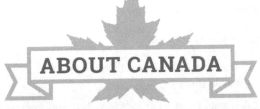

ABOUT CANADA

DENTAL CARE

Brandon Doucet

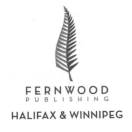

FERNWOOD
PUBLISHING

HALIFAX & WINNIPEG

Development editor: Tanya Andrusieczko
Copyediting: Brenda Conroy
Design: John van der Woude
Printed and bound in Canada

Published by Fernwood Publishing
2970 Oxford Street, Halifax, Nova Scotia B3L 2W4
and 748 Broadway Avenue, Winnipeg, MB R3G 0X3
www.fernwoodpublishing.ca

Fernwood Publishing Company Limited gratefully acknowledges the financial support of the Government of Canada through the Canada Book Fund and the Canada Council for the Arts. We acknowledge the Province of Manitoba for support through the Manitoba Publishers Marketing Assistance Program and the Book Publishing Tax Credit. We acknowledge the Nova Scotia Department of Communities, Culture and Heritage for support through the Publishers Assistance Fund.

   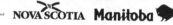

Library and Archives Canada Cataloguing in Publication
Title: Dental care / Brandon Doucet.
Names: Doucet, Brandon, author.
Series: About Canada (Black Point, N.S.)
Description: Series statement: About Canada | Includes bibliographical references and index.
Identifiers: Canadiana (print) 20220497923 | Canadiana (ebook) 20220497966 | ISBN 9781773635910 (softcover) | ISBN 9781773636122 (EPUB) | ISBN 9781773636139 (PDF)
Subjects: LCSH: Dental care—Canada. | LCSH: Dental economics—Canada. | LCSH: Dentistry—Canada.
Classification: LCC RK52.4.C3 D68 2023 | DDC 362.197600971—dc23

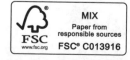

CONTENTS

"Those in power can kill one, two, or three roses,
but they will never be able to stop the coming of spring."
— *President of Brazil Lula da Silva's historic speech, April 7, 2018*

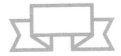

ABBREVIATIONS

CDA	Canadian Dental Association
CDSS	College of Dental Surgeons of Saskatchewan
CCF	Co-operative Commonwealth Federation
CFNU	Canadian Federation of Nurses Unions
CLHIA	Canadian Life and Health Insurance Association
CHA	Canada Health Act
CMA	Canadian Medical Association
CSC	Correctional Services Canada
CWF	community water fluoridation
DCC	Dental Corporation of Canada
DND	Department of National Defence
DSO	dental service organization
IFHP	Interim Federal Health Program
NHS	National Health Service (UK)
NIHB	Non-Insured Health Benefits
PBO	Parliamentary Budget Officer
RAMQ	Régie de l'assurance maladie du Québec
SDC	SmileDirectClub
SDP	Saskatchewan Dental Plan
SID	supplier-induced demand

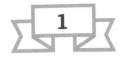

THE STRUGGLE FOR ORAL HEALTH

Several components contribute to poor oral health, with the most obvious being dental decay, also known as cavities, or caries. Dental decay occurs when bacteria in the mouth digest sugars and produce an acid byproduct that demineralizes the teeth. Once demineralization undermines enough tooth structure, a hole forms in the tooth. If left untreated, the cavity will continue to grow. Over the centuries, access to sugar has changed trends in dental decay. In the nineteenth century, sugar was a commodity of the affluent, who developed cavities at disproportionately higher rates as a result. Nowadays, sugar is widely and cheaply available, and dental decay disproportionately affects those of low socioeconomic status.[1]

Another component of poor oral health is gum disease, also known as periodontal disease. Gum disease is caused by the bacteria in the plaque on the teeth producing byproducts that cause inflammation of the gums and eventually the supporting bone underneath. Over time inflammation leads to the destruction of tissue, which is what most would see as their gums receding. If enough supporting tissue is destroyed by this process, pain and mobility issues can cause the teeth to lose their ability to function.[2] Globally, untreated dental decay is the most common health condition, and severe periodontal disease is the sixth most common.[3]

Oral health also encompasses the ability to chew, which we need in order to eat and properly digest food.[4] Cancers can impact oral health by damaging the tissues and supporting structures of the mouth, and misaligned teeth can affect both chewing efficiency and a person's willingness to smile.[5] Being able to speak and smile are components of oral health that can have profound social consequences; for people who have lost teeth, adequate replacement can restore the ability to chew and speak, and the confidence to smile.

Despite the critical importance of good oral health, which is highlighted throughout this chapter, our society tends to consider the perfect smile as a sign of status.[6] People make assumptions about individuals baring a smile with misaligned, broken, discoloured and missing teeth in comparison to someone whose teeth are perfectly straight and white. Studies have shown that people see those with a perfect smile as more intelligent, successful and attractive than those whose smile shows visible decay.[7]

There is a tacit acknowledgement in this line of thinking that access to dental care and good oral health are determined by one's income. This is borne out by the evidence, as oral health outcomes are consistently worse for people of a lower socioeconomic status. A study using data from the Canadian Health Measures Survey (2007–09) found that the prevalence of decayed and missing teeth and the prevalence of oral pain all decreased as income increased.[8] The presence of periodontal disease in adults increased as education levels decreased.[9] People who avoided the dentist due to cost were three and a half times more likely to have untreated dental decay than the group that did not avoid the dentist due to cost.[10] People in the lowest income quintile were shown to be seven times more likely to be missing all of their teeth than those in the highest income quintile.[11] People in the lower income quintiles experience a greater burden of dental disease and face greater difficulties accessing care, which results in more teeth deteriorating until they are no longer salvageable or are too costly to save.

Financial barriers inhibit people from accessing dental care, and the more income a person has, the more likely they are to have dental insurance and disposable income to pay for care out of pocket.[12] While other factors, such as diet, oral hygiene, alcohol and tobacco use influence oral health, socioeconomic status remains the most important.[13] The goal of improving access to dental care for Canadians should be paired with a plan to end poverty, something that should not be difficult in such a rich country but nevertheless is beyond the scope of this book.[14] This book focuses on access to dental care. This is not to downplay the importance of the other factors but rather to highlight the greatest factor that contributes to inequality in oral health outcomes.

In 2014, the Canadian Academy of Health Sciences sought to understand the differences in oral health outcomes between low- and high-income groups. When factors like dental decay, dental pain and difficulty eating food were examined, it was found that 90–95 percent of the differences between the income groups could be accounted for by access to dental care and socioeconomic status. Access to dental care accounted for over 50 percent of the differences between income groups for dental decay and difficulty eating, and it was a close second to socioeconomic status for dental pain. Oral health behaviours accounted for the remaining 5–10 percent for each category.[15] Clearly, lacking access to dental care leads to worse oral health outcomes.

Since access to dental care is an essential component of achieving good oral health, it is worth exploring what factors influence it. The two largest factors contributing to access to dental care are socioeconomic status and geography.[16] Socioeconomic status influences the likelihood of having dental insurance and disposable income to pay for care. In terms of geography, a disproportionate number of dental professionals practise in urban centres, leaving many rural communities underserviced.[17] Too few dental providers results in a dental workforce that is unable to meet the population needs, which results in rationing of services and people having to travel greater distances to find the nearest dental office.

Geography and socioeconomic status are compounding factors, and people with low incomes in rural or remote communities tend to have worse oral health than those who experience only one of those factors.[18] Taken together with colonial policies of underfunding healthcare, high food costs and lack of access to clean drinking water are significant factors for why many Indigenous communities struggle with achieving good oral health.[19]

Other factors also influence access to dental care. For example, people with disabilities may require specific equipment or sedation in order to access care, but these are not widely available.[20] Language and cultural practices can also influence access.[21] Injustices can lead to mistrust in the dental profession, which can cause hesitancy in seeking care. This is particularly true for Indigenous Peoples, who faced particularly inhumane dental treatment in the residential school system.[22] Clearly, access to dental care is made worse by colonialism, ableism and racism. Structures of social and economic inequality affect oral health, and the struggle for dental care is an important part of broader struggles for justice.

Without access to comprehensive dental care, people tend to

ration dental services, which can take different forms. For some, it is skipping a cleaning. For others, it means extracting a tooth instead of saving it with root canal treatment. For others, it means living with decayed and infected teeth for many years. Preventative services and early interventions are neglected, and dental disease festers, which leads to pain and infection.[23]

ORAL HEALTH AND OVERALL HEALTH

While historically and politically, the mouth has been treated as separate from the body, evidence is mounting that poor oral health has significant downstream effects on an individual's overall health.[24] As highlighted by Dr. Hasan Sheikh from the Canadian Association of Emergency Physicians, poor oral health has been associated with cardiovascular disease, diabetes, having a low-birth-weight infant, aspiration pneumonia, erectile dysfunction, osteoporosis, metabolic syndrome and stroke.[25] Recent research has found that people with active gum disease have a higher likelihood of being hospitalized or dying from COVID-19 than people with good oral health.[26]

Some studies show that poor oral health is not just associated with poorer general health but can actually cause it. For example, the provision of regular oral care in long-term care settings has been shown to reduce residents' risk for aspiration pneumonia.[27] This lung infection can be caused by bacteria being inhaled from the significant plaque buildup on the teeth.

A bidirectional relationship between oral health and type II diabetes has been identified. Treatment of periodontal disease in type II diabetics leads to improved blood sugar control equivalent to adding a new medication.[28] Conversely, individuals with poorly controlled type II diabetes experience more severe periodontal disease.[29] Treating periodontal disease has also been shown to reduce patients' risk for cardiovascular disease.[30] Periodontal disease leads to chronic inflammation, which worsens both type II diabetes and cardiovascular disease.

Poor oral health also has mental-health related consequences. A study from Cambridge University determined that "tooth loss causally increased depression among US adults. Losing ten or more teeth had an impact comparable to adults with major depressive disorder not receiving antidepressant drugs."[31] Poor oral health has been shown to negatively impact a person's self-esteem and affect the quality of their social interactions.[32]

Lack of access to dental care contributes considerably to the cycle of poverty. First, without dental insurance or sufficient disposable income, and consequently insufficient access to dental care, many experience poor oral health. Poor oral health can affect employability, further perpetuating the cycle of poverty.[33] One can imagine the preconceived notions an employer might have of an individual at a job interview who has visible dental decay or missing front teeth. Further, dental pain may impact a person's performance at work; it can be challenging to concentrate on tasks while experiencing significant discomfort, especially if the same ache has negatively impacted quality of sleep. In the time an individual lacks access to dental care, dental disease only worsens, further exacerbating the problem.

Conversely, oral health treatment can have considerable positive effects. For instance, individuals undergoing treatment for addiction who were provided with dental care were more likely to find employment and abstain from drug use and less likely to experience homelessness when compared to their counterparts who did not receive dental treatment.[34] In other words, access to dental care is an important factor in breaking the cycle of poverty.

Oral health is also relevant to overall health insofar as it impacts a person's ability to chew efficiently, which is critical to attaining proper nutrition and digestion. People who cannot chew tend to eat softer and less healthy food. In 2018, the Public Health Agency of Canada estimated that 1.8 million Canadians were unable to chew. The report identified that the main causes of the inability to chew were 1) decayed or painful teeth; 2) no dentures or poorly fitting dentures; and 3) medical conditions (e.g., Parkinson's disease).[35] The report demonstrated a class divide relating to the ability to chew. For instance, those of low socioeconomic status were often unable to get their teeth extracted, were unable to afford dentures to replace their extracted teeth or had old dentures that no longer fit. As a result, many people were forced to live with decayed teeth for years. When the pain becomes unbearable, many incur debt to access the necessary treatment.

The report identified that adults who have a permanent disability leaving them unable to work were four times more likely to be unable to chew when compared to people who are employed. Further, those with less than a high school education were three times more likely to be unable to chew than those with university degrees. Those in the lowest income quintile were more than three times more likely to be unable to chew than those in the top income quintile, who were more likely to access to dental care.

Clearly oral health is more than just having the perfect smile. A comprehensive view of oral health and how it interacts with overall health should guide how governments fund and deliver dental care. The World Health Organization states that universal health coverage should be a global priority and that oral health treatment should be integrated into healthcare.[36] The World Dental Federation defines oral health as "multi-faceted and includes the ability to speak, smile, smell, taste, touch, chew, swallow and convey a range of emotions though facial expressions with confidence and without pain, discomfort and disease of the craniofacial complex (head, face, and oral cavity)."[37] Given the importance of oral health and its relationship to overall health, the aim of this book is to highlight how Canada's current dental care system is inconsistent with the primary purpose of the Canada Health Act, which is "to protect, promote and restore the physical and mental well-being of residents of Canada and to facilitate reasonable access to health services without financial or other barriers."[38]

ORAL HEALTH AND CANADA'S HEALTHCARE SYSTEM

Poor oral health negatively affects individuals and the broader society. In Canada, where large numbers of people lack access to dental care, people suffer poorer oral health and consequently poorer general health. Thus, poor oral health increases the need for spending on general healthcare. While comprehensive estimates of the increased healthcare costs due to lack of access to dental care have not been done due to the complexity of analysis, some studies have narrowed in on direct and quantifiable effects of poor access to dental care. For instance, many people who cannot afford emergency dental care end up in doctors' offices and emergency departments seeking pain relief for a toothache.[39] While physicians and nurse practitioners try to help individuals suffering with immense dental pain, they do not have the necessary skills or equipment to address dental issues.

The most common reason people go to a physician for dental pain is a dental abscess. An abscess occurs most often when a cavity reaches the nerve inside of a tooth, causing a toothache and infection. This infection leads to pus collecting around the tip of the root of the tooth, which causes the face to swell. Anyone who has experienced a toothache knows just how miserable this is, leading people without access to dental care to seek relief wherever they can. Some even try to extract their own teeth in a desperate attempt to get out of pain.[40]

A study from the Ontario Oral Health Alliance showed just how frequent visits to physicians for dental pain are. In 2014, Ontario emergency rooms were visited 61,000 times and physicians' offices were visited 222,000 times by patients seeking treatment for dental pain. That amounted to one visit every three minutes to a medical clinic and one visit every nine minutes to an ER by patients.[41] One study showed that ER visits for dental pain increased more than population growth between 2001and 2015 in Ontario, which is an indicator that access to dental care has been worsening.[42] A study in British Columbia found that 1 percent of all visits to the emergency department were for patients with non-traumatic dental pain caused by decay.[43] However, physicians are not trained to extract teeth or perform root canal treatments to deal with dental abscesses, so they can only offer Band-Aid relief in the form of a prescription for antibiotics and/or pain medications. Nationwide, this problem is estimated to cost taxpayers more than $150 million per year.[44] This number is likely an underestimate as it looks at the minimum cost per visit to the emergency department for dental pain, when in reality some people need to be hospitalized, which is much more expensive. Despite these resources being used to help people with dental pain, patients are still left needing to see a dentist. This inefficiency could be eliminated if everyone had access dental and primary preventative care in the first place.

A dental abscess is a localized infection, but if left untreated or treated improperly, the infection can spread to other parts of the body. An infection of an upper tooth can spread to the brain, while an infection of a lower tooth can cause swelling and compression of the airway.[45] For people with specific heart conditions, bacteria from a dental infection can spread to the inner lining of the heart.[46] The spread of a dental infection in these ways can become fatal.

In 2015, a nine-year-old girl in Edmonton fell gravely ill from malnutrition, septic shock and congestive heart failure caused by a dental infection.[47] In 2016, a man in his 30s had a dental infection that led to sepsis and resulted in him losing his right leg below his knee, the fingers on his left hand and several toes on his left foot. He was in a medically induced coma for a week and a half, followed by over a month in the intensive care unit, where he required dialysis for his kidneys, followed by a year in a long-term care setting.[48] In June 2021, a person from Sioux Lookout died from a dental infection that led to sepsis as the tooth was left untreated due to lack of access to dental care.[49] While these stories occasionally make the news headlines, undoubtedly many others are not reported.

In a country with universal healthcare, these people are able access a health provider and treatment, but not the right kind of treatment at the right time from the right provider.[50] The healthcare system uses tremendous resources to react to a problem that could have easily been prevented with upstream investments in public dental care at a fraction of the cost. This represents a serious shortcoming of Canada's healthcare system: it reacts to health problems rather than proactively preventing problems from happening in the first place.

The inability of people with dental pain to see the right provider results in suboptimal treatment for their condition, which has its own consequences. Patients are often given two prescriptions when they present to a physician for dental pain, one for an antibiotic and another for pain medication, which due to the severity of a toothache often comes in the form of an opioid.[51] There are consequences of being over-reliant on these two types of medications, especially considering that they would usually not be needed if the person had been able to seek expedient and proper treatment from a dentist.

Antibiotics kill or inhibit the growth of bacteria, which is useful when fighting an infection. It is important that we use antibiotics sparingly though, as bacteria can learn to survive repeat exposures to antibiotics, which results in strains of bacteria that are resistant to the drug. When someone seeks treatment for a dental infection from a physician, they are given an antibiotic, but the underlying infected tooth is left in place until the patient seeks treatment from a dentist. This often leads to the infected tooth flaring up again down the road, as many seeking this type of treatment are unable to afford the subsequent dental care. In most cases, patients could have had the infected tooth extracted without needing an antibiotic. This overuse of antibiotics without any clinical benefit gives bacteria an opportunity to develop resistance.

In 2019, it was estimated that drug-resistant diseases kill 1.27 million people worldwide each year.[52] A report from the government of the United Kingdom stated that on our current trajectory this number could balloon to 10 million per year in 2050.[53] The complications associated with antibiotic resistant infections are expensive to treat and thus siphon resources away from other health services. We need to stop over-relying on antibiotics in Canada as a substitute for proper access to dental care, and thus lessen the number of antibiotic resistant infections in the process.

When patients go to their physician for the treatment of a dental abscess, they are also often given pain medication. Due to the severity of pain a toothache causes, an opioid is often needed.[54] Opioids are highly addictive and should be used sparingly. Rather than masking dental pain with opioids, it is wiser to treat the root cause of the pain by ensuring patients can access dental care. With proper access to dental care for all, many of these emergencies could have been prevented.

When children suffer from poor oral health and lack of access to dental care, they often need general anesthetic in a hospital setting to be treated. This not only creates traumatic experiences for children, but it also places an increased strain on the healthcare system. Cavities are the leading cause of day surgery for children aged one to five, accounting for approximately one in three day surgeries in this age range.[55] There are significant regional differences across the country, with children in rural communities needing dental surgery three times more often than their urban counterparts. Similarly, children from low-income families are more than three times more likely to need dental surgery than their high-income counterparts. Children from communities with a high proportion of Indigenous People were in need of dental surgery at rates approximately eight times greater than children from communities with a low proportion of Indigenous People.

This situation was made worse by the COVID-19 pandemic as many rural communities rely on dentists who fly into the community to treat patients. With travel restrictions on top of an already limited number of dentists working in these communities, the waitlist in Nunavut doubled for children's dental surgery, and children's health suffered as a consequence. In 2021, Nunavut, a territory with a population of only 38,700, had 1,000 children on the waitlist for dental surgery.[56]

With dental day surgeries costing on average $1,564 per child in Canada, it is far more expensive to allow dental disease to fester until children need general anesthesia in a hospital setting to be treated.[57] The problem is that many children are unable to access dental care until the decay is so extensive that the child could not tolerate the dental work while conscious. If children were able to easily access preventative and restorative dental care, as well as a healthy diet, many of these dental surgeries could be avoided.

Dental surgeries in children are a sign of rampant dental decay leading to pain and infection.[58] This suffering can affect a child's ability to eat and sleep, which can have lifelong ramifications. Nutritional deficiencies and lack of sleep can result in failure to thrive and have long-term impacts on the development of the nervous system.[59] A woman in Nunavut spoke to the CBC about her 12-year-old son losing 15 pounds while waiting to have a tooth removed.[60]

Access to dental care is also important for the detection of certain medical conditions. The human immunodeficiency virus (HIV) can cause sores in the mouth that can be detected by a dental professional, which would result in the patient being referred to a physician for further investigation. Eating disorders and acid reflux can be indicated if there is erosion of the outer enamel layer of teeth.[61] Signs of undiagnosed diabetes and hypertension can be detected during dental visits, and early detection of cancers of the throat and mouth can lead to greater survival rates.[62] Those who lack access to routine dental care do not have a dental professional regularly looking out for these signs and are more likely to have these conditions diagnosed at a later stage in the disease's progression. Later detection of these conditions ultimately leads to greater healthcare spending and worse outcomes for individuals.

The effects of poor oral health extend to individuals, the healthcare system and the broader society. Too often, discussions around addressing access to dental care focus solely on the immediate cost to governments of funding a dental plan, but it ignores the broader effects that poor oral health have on our society and the suffering it causes to individuals.

2

THE STRUCTURE OF DENTAL CARE

Medicare, the universal healthcare system in Canada, is considered a boon to its citizens.[1] Medicare is not one healthcare program but is rather 13 different provincial and territorial health insurance programs tied together by national standards that the jurisdictions must meet in order to receive federal funding. Nevertheless, the promise of Medicare is that if a person is sick, they will be helped regardless of their financial status. While this may be true for physician services, many other essential health-related services, including dentistry, prescription drugs and vision and auditory care among others, have been excluded from the universal coverage of Medicare, relegated instead to the private market.

The exclusion of dental care from Canada's universal healthcare system means that provincial and territorial governments, the jurisdictions responsible for healthcare, do not guarantee dental insurance for everyone.[2] The majority of people access dental care in the private market, either through private insurance or out-of-pocket payments. Private dental spending accounted for a staggering 94 percent of the $15 billion spent on dental care in 2017.[3] Of the private dental spending, about 60 percent comes from private insurance and 40 percent comes from out-of-pocket payments.

Private dental insurance is usually provided as part of a benefits package tied to a person's employment, and the delivery of dental care occurs primarily in private practices. Both the private practices and insurance companies have a fiduciary responsibility to maximize profits, and this drive for profits directly results in our society's most vulnerable being left behind. Only 6 percent of dental spending comes from targeted government programs that go towards marginalized populations (e.g., children, social assistance recipients, Indigenous Peoples).[4] The tiny proportion of dental spending that is public is an important indicator as it is inversely correlated with the proportion of people who avoid the dentist due to financial constraints.[5]

While ranking among the highest in overall per capita dental spending, Canada ranks second last in its share of public dental spending in comparison to other countries in the Organization of Economic

Figure 2.1 Percentage of Private and Public Dental Spending in Canada in 2017

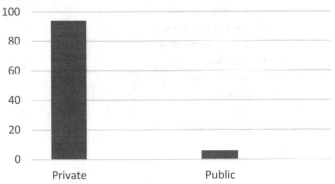

Source: Canadian Institute for Health Information, National Health Expenditure Trends, November 4, 2021, www.cihi.ca/en/national-health-expenditure-trends.

Co-operation and Development.[6,] Even in the United States, public dental spending accounts for 10 percent of dental spending, and Canada is far behind Germany and Japan, which have public dental spending rates of 58 and 78 percent, respectively.[7]

Figure 2.2 Percentage of Public Dental Spending as a Share of Total Dental Spending

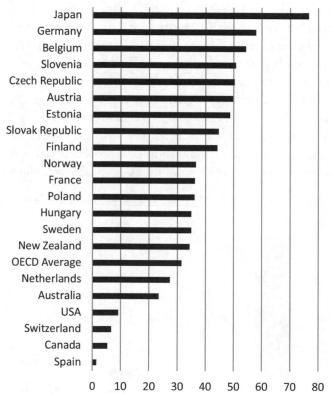

Source: Marion Devaux, "Income-related inequalities in health care services utilization in 18 selected OECD countries," European Journal of Health Economics, 2015 Jan;16, 1: 21–33. doi: 10.1007/ s10198-013-0546-4.

Canada has not always performed quite so poorly when it comes to the share of public dental spending. In the years after the implementation of universal healthcare, there were increases in both public and private dental spending. By 1980, public spending hovered around 20 percent of total dental spending, but since then, it has steadily declined to its current 6 percent.[8]

In 2018, more than one in three (35.4 percent) Canadians had no dental insurance,[9] meaning they paid the full cost of dental care out of pocket and thus were more likely to seek treatment only for emergencies, rather than accessing preventative care and early intervention.[10] This was emphasized by a survey done by Ipsos Reid and the Canadian Dental Association which found that "only 29% of Canadians agree unequivocally that they would still get regular check-ups from a dentist if they didn't have a dental plan."[11]

Since accessing dental care in Canada relies so heavily on private payment and private delivery, resources are allocated differently than in the publicly funded healthcare system, which is free at the point of access. People who reported having poor general health in Canada were more than twice as likely to seek medical treatment than those who reported having excellent health. In contrast, those who reported poor oral health were half as likely to seek dental care than those who reported excellent oral health.[12]

In 2017, Statistics Canada found that 22.8 percent of the population, or 6.8 million people, avoided the dentist due to financial constraints.[13] The lack of access to dental care in Canada is a by-product of how the system is structured. Understanding the driving forces of profit-making that are embedded in private funding and delivery of dental care shines a light on how our society's most vulnerable become disenfranchised.

PRIVATE HEALTH INSURANCE

Since dental, vision and auditory care and prescription drugs were excluded from the newly implemented healthcare system, people began searching for ways to more reliably access these services. As a result, the market for private health insurance in Canada greatly increased in the years after Medicare was introduced.[14] Other factors that helped translate this increased demand into more business for insurance companies included the labour movement championing the inclusion of dental insurance in collective bargaining agreements[15] and the state introducing tax incentives that allowed employers to deduct their contributions to their employee's dental insurance from business income. These factors led to an increase in the number of people who had employer-sponsored insurance. Since more people could access dental care with these plans, private dental spending rose significantly in the years after universal healthcare was implemented.[16]

From the perspective of insurance companies, it was beneficial to provide insurance to union members because the companies saw the large numbers of people involved as an opportunity to mitigate risk.[17] Insurance companies know that the risk will be lower on average when providing insurance to large groups of people, because the risk of people with high dental needs is spread out amongst the group. By contrast, people who buy dental insurance individually are likely doing so because they need dental (and other) care, which makes these people on average a higher risk and less profitable.[18]

Insurance companies also use other techniques to mitigate risk and thus decrease the amounts they pay out — and increase their profits. The first technique is a copayment, a percentage of the dentist's fee that a patient must pay out of pocket, and this tends to be higher for more expensive procedures. The second technique is requiring prior approval for more expensive procedures, which can often take several weeks, slowing and deterring patients from receiving those treatments. If an insured patient has a toothache, they might either save the tooth with the more expensive root canal but have to wait a month for the prior approval to see how much will be covered, or they could relieve their pain instantly by having the cheaper extraction. The third technique insurance companies use are deductibles, an amount of money a person must pay out of pocket each year before the insurance plan will start paying anything. Fourth, insurance companies reduce risk by placing yearly limits on the amount they will pay out. If someone needs dental work above that amount in a given year, they are expected to pay the full amount themselves. Lastly, insurance plans can choose not to cover certain procedures.[19] Insurance companies' risk mitigation strategies can deter a patient from going to the dentist at all, which is beneficial to the insurance company, but harmful to the person in need of dental care. In Canada, there are no minimum standards for dental insurance, so the quality of coverage varies widely based on what the employer is willing to pay.[20] As a consequence, many people who have dental insurance still struggle accessing care.[21]

Dental insurance is also precarious: when tied to employment, coverage is jeopardized when a person loses a job or retires; and when tied to relationship status, spousal benefits are terminated when a relationship ends. With declining unionization rates, dental insurance is also harder to come by; a 2022 study in the Waterloo Region in Ontario found that full-time, low-income workers were 56 percent less likely to have dental insurance than they were a decade ago.[22] The rise of the precarious "gig economy," where benefits like dental insurance are not tied to labour, has undoubtedly contributed to this, but also many conventional jobs that once provided these benefits are no longer doing so. This has led to a rising number of people without dental insurance and access to dental care.[23] The financial downturn sparked by the COVID-19 pandemic has only made things worse.

Canada's universal healthcare system is a good example of how to alleviate the instability of work-related insurance. In Canada, medical insurance is not tied to employment, so it is constant, even in economic downturns. The same is not true for dental care, as people access these services primarily through their work-related plans and secondarily through out-of-pocket payments. When people become unemployed, they also lose disposable income to pay for care. This shows how foundational Canada's universal healthcare system is and how flawed it is to rely on work-related insurance for essential health services like dental care.

If Canada continues on its current trajectory, the number of people with private health insurance will continue to decrease. This factor, along with a lack of sizeable investments in public dental programs, will result in Canada continuing to be an outlier amongst developed nations when it comes to inequalities in access to dental care. It has been demonstrated how poor oral health affects individuals as well as the societies they live in. Yet, the problems associated with poor oral health are not inevitable; they are a consequence of policy decisions. The for-profit nature of dental insurance creates incentives to push greater costs onto patients, deny coverage for necessary procedures and neglect those of low socioeconomic status and those with high dental needs. For-profit dental insurance is not consistent with a dental care system that allocates resources based on need but rather one based on the ability to pay.

PRIVATE PRACTICE

If private dental insurance is one of the main components that shapes how Canadians access dental care, the other is private practice.[24] A private practice is a dental clinic that is owned by a dental professional, a group of investors or some combination thereof.[25] In some jurisdictions, dental hygienists can set up their own private practice independent of a dentist.[26] All provinces allow denturists, who are dental professionals who provide denture care directly to patients, to set up their own independent private practice.[27] Both dental hygienists and denturists have long fought for the right to have private practices independent of dentists.[28] Despite this, the ownership of private practices by dentists and group investors remains the dominant form in Canada.[29]

The owners of private-practice dental clinics need to run the clinic by hiring staff and maintaining the building and equipment among other responsibilities, and in return the owners seek to make a profit, just like any other business owners. Dentists who do not own the dental clinic are referred to as associates.

Both the owner and associate dentists make money through their provision of dental services to patients. Owners have the added income from the clinic after all the bills and staff are paid. Dentists tend to be paid a percentage of their collections from the dental procedures they perform, with the percentage of collections varying with factors like geography.[30] For example, recruiting dentists to rural areas is more difficult, and increasing the percentage of collections is one way of overcoming this. The collections are determined by how much of the billings to patients and insurance companies are actually received by the clinic. In order for dentists to earn an income they deem worthwhile, they must bill an average amount per day and ensure those bills are being paid.

In Canada, the minority of dentists who work in federal prisons, hospitals and academia are salaried, but the overwhelming majority of dentists bill patients on a fee-for-service basis, which means that patients are charged a fee for each procedure that is performed. Each procedure has a fee that is recommended by provincial dental associations in their annual fee guides, though these fee guides do not need to be followed.[31] Often, general dentists will follow the fee guide, as this is what insurance companies tend to follow. Specialists have their own fee guides, with the fees being higher and having more variation.[32] The fee guide includes uncommon procedures with independent consideration, meaning the dentist must determine what they think is reasonable to charge.

Provincial dental associations, which represent and are composed primarily of dentists, determine fees by what they perceive to be the cost of doing business. Though they do not release their exact calculations, provincial dental associations consider factors like the amount of time needed for a procedure, as well as the cost of supplies, owning an office and paying staff, along with what they see to be a reasonable rate of return.[33]

The exception to the provincial dental fee guides was Alberta from 1997 to 2018, when the provincial dental association did not release a recommended fee guide.[34] This led to Alberta patients paying more for services than in any other province. A review done by the Alberta NDP in 2016 found that "the average costs of nearly 50 procedures are 44 per cent higher in Alberta than in British Columbia, 38 per cent more than in Saskatchewan and 25 per cent more than in Ontario."[35] Eventually a recommended fee guide was put in place, but Alberta's dental fees remain the highest in the country and the fee guide is only a suggestion.[36]

Dental fees have risen on average higher than inflation since the late 1990s.[37] An Ontario study found that from 2001 to 2020, dental fees rose 81 percent while inflation overall rose by 41 percent.[38] Many insured people do not notice this rise as their insurance covers most of the cost at the time of the appointment, but they are still footing the bill through their insurance premiums and higher out-of-pocket expenses.

Paying dentists on a fee-for-service basis leads to the potential problem of overtreatment as the more services that are provided, the more the dentist can bill.[39] Dentistry also lacks standardization of diagnosis and treatment planning, which leads to the decisions in dentistry being less scientifically based than in medicine.[40] The combination of these factors creates a space where it is difficult to figure out whether overtreatment is occurring. This is problematic as patients are in a vulnerable position when they visit the dentist, as Blomqvist and Woolley from the CD Howe Institute explain:

> Clearly, there is information asymmetry of this kind in the market for dental care as well. Buyers of dental services are disadvantaged by their lack of professional expertise not only when it comes to deciding which provider to choose, but also with respect to what treatment approaches they should opt for when they have oral health problems.[41]

Due to the information asymmetry between dentists and their patients, it is crucial that patients trust their dental provider's recommendations. If patients are skeptical of a dentist's recommendations and do not follow through with all of the treatment plan, they may be avoiding overtreatment, but they can also be avoiding necessary care. A 2009 poll conducted by Ipsos Reid in partnership with the Canadian Dental Association found that more people see dentists as businesspeople than as doctors.[42] This shows that there is no consensus amongst the population that dentists are looking out for the public's best interests.

In economic terms, overtreatment is what is known as supplier-induced demand (SID).[43] This is because a dentist can manipulate their patients in order to justify performing more procedures. But overtreatment can also be caused by dentists who genuinely believe in a more aggressive approach to things like diagnosing cavities, despite not being backed up by scientific evidence. In between these two approaches are gray areas that can be difficult to discern. But the patient is receiving unnecessary treatment either way.

Unfortunately, the literature on SID in dentistry in Canada is limited.[44] Research in the United Kingdom found that the fee-for-service model in dentistry led to SID.[45] A study in Taiwan found increased frequencies of dental visits in places with a greater concentration of dentists.[46] Research has also found that the fee-for-service model leads to increased spending when compared to a salaried approach.[47]

A 2020 survey of dentists in Canada asked for their treatment recommendations for various clinical situations; the recommendations ranged from very conservative to very aggressive, with the latter creating more opportunities to bill patients. The dentists were also asked questions about their views and professional situation. The study found that dentists who described themselves as businesspeople were on average more aggressive in their treatment approach than their colleagues who described themselves as healthcare providers. Other factors associated with a more aggressive treatment approach were an income over $250,000 per year, being unsatisfied with how busy your schedule is and still having student loans.[48] This is concerning as treatment recommendations should not be influenced by these outside factors, but rather on scientific evidence.

Another study showed how financial considerations can subconsciously affect a dentist's treatment recommendations. The researchers showed dentists a decayed tooth that was borderline savable with a root canal treatment, or otherwise it would need to be extracted and the tooth replaced with a dental implant. The study found that dentists who placed implants were more likely to say the tooth should be extracted and an implant placed, whereas dentists who did root canal treatments were more likely to recommend saving the tooth.[49] This means that the surveyed dentists were more likely to recommend a treatment they could profit from. While these biases may be subconscious, it is nevertheless worrying.

While the evidence from quantitative studies on SID hold more weight, anecdotal evidence can help paint the picture of real-life scenarios. An episode of CBC *Marketplace* in 2012 called "Is Your Dentist Ripping You Off?" demonstrated some disturbing trends.[50] A CBC researcher, Theresa, received two checkups from faculty members at the University of Toronto's dental school as a baseline and subsequently went to 20 different dental offices for treatment plans. The control exams only recommended several cleanings and possibly a crown, but the combined results of the 20 other plans was treatment recommendations for 19 of her teeth: fillings on teeth without cavities, a few root canals, cosmetic veneers on her six front teeth and even two replacements for a bridge that other dentists told her looked great. While many dentists recommended treatment plans for Theresa that were similar to the control exams, many did not. The inconsistencies in recommended treatment plans had costs that varied from $144 to $11,931.[51]

Some dentists recommend replacing "old metal fillings" with tooth-coloured fillings. This sales technique preys on patients' fear of mercury in the metal amalgam fillings and the information asymmetry between dentists and patients. The reality is that amalgam fillings are safe, with the mercury beng locked inside the fillings, and do not need to be replaced unless a cavity forms or the tooth fractures.[52]

Private practice has also seen an increase in treatments for cosmetic dentistry since the 1980s, a time when the number of dentists increased and community water fluoridation and better oral hygiene led to significant improvements in oral health.[53] In 2009, responding to Ipsos Reid poll findings, the Canadian Dental Association concluded: "Many people assume that the cosmetic side of the profession is largely driven by dentists looking for revenue and is, therefore, not really about patient health or well-being."[54] Patients need to rely on the dentist's judgement: the aggressive marketing of cosmetic dentistry takes advantage of this trust, as patients struggle to discern between what is necessary and what is cosmetic.

Veneers are one of the dental procedures that have become much more prevalent during the rise of cosmetic dentistry. Veneers are a staple of Hollywood-smile makeovers that allow patients to change the shape and colour of their front teeth by shaving down the outer layer of enamel and replacing it with a custom-made porcelain or composite covering. While this may result in the desired esthetic outcome, it requires the removal of healthy tooth structure and requires lifelong maintenance.[55] The decision to have dental veneers should not be taken lightly as it is a decision that one can come to regret. The aggressive marketing of veneers by dentists increases this chance, as some dentists recommend veneers to their patients unprompted.[56] Even Dr. Gordon Christenson, a US dentist and leader for decades in the fields of continuing dental education and cosmetic dentistry, sounded the alarm in 2003: "I was one of the original instigators of the recognition of esthetic dentistry, over 25 years ago. However, my pet subject has turned into a monster with unbelievable overtreatment of unsuspecting patients. The problem of overtreatment is not limited to esthetic dentistry. It is spread throughout the profession."[57] Dentistry in Canada and the US is highly integrated, and overtreatment has not been addressed in either jurisdiction.

Considering some of the concerning trends in dentistry in Canada, it is worth looking into how dentists are governed and disciplined. Dentists in Canada are self-regulating, meaning the oversight of the profession is managed by dentists. Important responsibilities that are delegated in self-regulation are the ability to choose who can practise in the profession and what standards the people in the profession must conform to, and ensuring ethical behaviour in professional practice.[58]

In Canada, each province and territory has its own dental board, which is composed primarily of dentists and is granted the responsibility of licensing and disciplining dentists.[59] The provincial dental board differs from the dental associations, as the board is meant to represent the public, whereas the associations represent dentists. While some argue that only dentists know the field well enough to govern the conduct of the profession, others argue that it is a conflict of interest to be responsible for disciplining your colleagues.[60]

As explained by Tracey Adams in *Regulating Professions*, in countries where self-regulating professions are present, such as the United Kingdom, the United States and Australia, the public tends to have a much harsher view of those professions: "Self-regulation is cast as an outdated practice that contributed to elitism and high prices, restricted competition, and led to excesses and abuses."[61]

Many examples have been found of self-regulating professions using their positions of power to close off access to the profession in order "to regulate market conditions in their favour, in the face of competition."[62] This is known as social closure and can help people understand the shortcomings of having members of a self-regulating profession be responsible for the public good. The story of dental therapy in Canada, discussed in the next chapter, is a great example of how social closure applies to dentistry.

Dentists, through the provincial dental boards, have tried looking out for the public good, but their approach is limited by their need to uphold and protect the image and system where private practice dentists are the beneficiaries. In order to seriously protect the public, the dental profession needs to address overtreatment and the lack of standardization in dentistry. But in confronting these issues, the self-regulating profession would need to harm their own image. The dental profession has a vested interest in maintaining their image, and that takes precedent over the public good.[63]

In 2018 in British Columbia, the Cayton report, which investigated professional health colleges, placed emphasis on the provincial dental board and highlighted many of these problems:

> The current model of professional regulation will not be adequate to protect patients. … There is a lack of relentless focus on the safety of patients in many but not all of the current colleges. Their governance is insufficiently independent, lacking a competency framework, a way of managing skill mix or clear accountability to the public they serve.[64]

The report recommends a complete overhaul of how the dental and other health professions are regulated in order increase transparency and accountability.

This is not meant to demonize dentists but rather to understand the incentives in place in the current dental care system and the public's distrust of the dental profession. Only by taking those concerns seriously can trust be rebuilt. This includes the need for greater standardization of dental treatments that are guided by scientific evidence, but this will not occur while profit is the driving force. The funding and delivery of dental care in Canada is highly privatized, and this leads to significant inequalities in access to care. Both insurance companies and private practice dentists are looking out for their own self-interest, which is often harmful to public health. It is time to look back into the history of dental care to understand how Canada got to this point.

THE HISTORY OF DENTAL CARE IN CANADA

Dentistry in Upper and Lower Canada started as a trade, dominated by middle-class, white, Anglo-Saxon men from the United States. In the nineteenth century, dentists were known as barber surgeons, and they offered a wide array of services, such as haircuts, enemas, bloodletting and fixing and pulling teeth.[1]

Even for those fortunate enough to afford dental care in those days, it was not glamorous. The painful procedures were done without local anesthetic. Little was known about the cause of dental disease, and partial or complete tooth loss was common. Dentistry, therefore, focused mainly on extracting teeth and making dentures rather than the prevention of dental disease.[2]

At this time there was no formal education needed to practise dentistry, and many learned the skills as an apprentice. Barber surgeons worked in cities, as these were the only places with enough people who could afford their services. People in rural settings had to make do however they could. It was common for a farmer or gunsmith to offer to pull teeth, and some even made dentures.[3]

Many barber surgeons from well-off backgrounds did an apprenticeship for two to four years, often while taking some medical courses before practising independently. They categorized themselves as trained dentists, distinguishing themselves from the untrained ones.[4] This trend originated in the United States and created division among dental practitioners, with trained dentists actively disparaging their untrained counterparts.[5]

Trained dentists often accused untrained dentists of being unskilled, deceitful and dirty, despite many untrained dentists being equally proficient to their trained counterparts. While some dentists were unhygienic in handling instruments, lied in advertisements or lacked particular skills, these problems were prevalent among both trained and untrained dentists. Many trained dentists wanted to raise their income and status in society by transitioning dentistry from a trade to a learned profession, and removing untrained dentists was seen as a necessary step.[6]

Dentists wanted to transition dentistry from a trade to a learned profession as the public had greater respect for learned professions and were willing to pay more for their services. In the mid-nineteenth century, dentistry was increasingly becoming its own specialty rather than one of the services offered by barber surgeons. This helped develop the technical skills of the field, which was needed to legitimize dentistry as a learned profession.[7]

Governments would often grant learned professions self-regulatory status. This autonomy was attractive for both the dental profession and the government. Dentists had greater control, which they could use to help raise the status of the profession. From the government's standpoint, this status provided low-cost regulation of an important area of the economy, as regulatory boards are self-funding.[8]

Upon Confederation, trained dentists in many provinces banded together to convince Canada's new politicians of their legitimacy as a learned profession rather than a trade. They did so by formulating legislation that granted dentists self-regulatory control over the profession and seeking approval from provincial governments.[9] Dentistry became a self-regulated profession in Ontario and Quebec in 1868 and 1869, respectively. In fact, Ontario had the first legislation in the world specifically pertaining to the regulation of dentistry. In both provinces, organized dentistry was given vast powers over the profession. Other provinces followed before the turn of the century.[10]

At Confederation, trained dentists were mainly American or British white men who came from well-connected, wealthy backgrounds. Researchers have pointed out that the trained dentists in Ontario were "men of reputation and influence who knew how to work the levers of power."[11] These powerful men were able to make it illegal to practise dentistry without a licence, and they controlled who could get a licence. While the establishment of a formal licensing process was necessary in the development of the dental profession, it was done in an undemocratic fashion that sought to eliminate competition in order to increase prices.

Trained dentists were successful in persuading politicians about the need to eliminate untrained dentists, but they had greater trouble convincing the public. Many politicians came from wealthy families and were able to afford dental care, but most of the population had limited means. Many people sought dental care from people with no formal training because it was their only option. Untrained dentists tended to be cheaper, and rural areas often did not have trained dentists. Tracey Adams states in *A Dentist and a Gentleman*: "The Ontario public had little respect for dentists or dentistry, and they refused to limit their patronage to 'respectable,' educated dentists."[12] As a result, some untrained dentists were able to continue practising in rural parts of Canada until World War I.[13]

Although it took from the mid-nineteenth to the twentieth century, dentistry was increasingly being recognized as a learned profession, due in part to the first dental school in Canada opening at the University of Toronto in 1875.[14] A standardized training program was needed to show that dentistry required a formal education rather than just mechanical skills. In the early twentieth century, research showed the link between sugar and dental decay, which furthered the scientific foundation of dentistry.[15] With the discovery of local anesthetics, making dental procedures less painful, people were more likely to seek out dental services. Advertisements promoted the concept of the perfect smile as a sign of social success, which raised the importance of oral health while further engraining the stigma of having poor oral health. These factors resulted in oral health and dental care gaining prominence in the public consciousness, which also helped raise dentistry to a learned profession.

THE FIGHT FOR MEDICARE AND THE EXCLUSION OF DENTAL CARE

The transition to a learned profession allowed dentists to more effectively lobby for their best interests. A long-standing fear of the dental profession was the inclusion of dental care in a government funded universal healthcare plan. Their lobbying against this, along with other factors, resulted in dental care being excluded from Medicare in Canada.

The concept of universal healthcare in Canada gained footing during the Great Depression, when the economic collapse made people destitute. From 1929–33, the gross national expenditure (overall public and private spending) fell by 42 percent.[16] The distress and pain experienced during the Great Depression caused many to look to "radical solutions" to ease their suffering. For many years, politicians believed that the popularity of the concept of universal healthcare would wane as material conditions improved after the Great Depression. To their surprise, the public was still very keen on universal healthcare following World War II, when standards of living were improving.[17] In 1937, the federal government tasked the Royal Commission on Dominion-Provincial Relations to study how the federal and provincial governments could respond to the economic downturn. The Commission's 1940 report came up with solutions like pensions and unemployment insurance and also indicated its support of the federal government aiding provinces in funding a healthcare plan. The proposed plan included dental care.[18]

However, it was not until the 1960s that Saskatchewan's government applied the conclusions of the Commission's studies and began implementing a universal health insurance plan. In 1960, the Co-operative Commonwealth Federation (CCF), led by Tommy Douglas, won the Saskatchewan election with 42 percent of the popular vote and 37 out of 54 seats. This victory was seen as a strong mandate to implement a universal healthcare plan, the first of its kind in North America.[19]

Tommy Douglas and the CCF's vision for universal healthcare included all medically necessary services, including prescription drugs and dental, vision and hearing care among other services.[20] However, the mandate for the 1960 election was limited to physician services, with the intention to expand the program to include other services like dental care later. The decision to implement universal healthcare faced fierce resistance from physicians, and the CCF did not want to increase resistance from other professions, like dentists. [21]

The opposition to universal healthcare came from doctors and their provincial and federal medical associations, along with business interests.[22] In anticipation of the Saskatchewan CCF's implementation of universal healthcare, the Canadian Medical Association (CMA) lobbied the federal Progressive Conservatives (PCs), under the leadership of John Diefenbaker, to study the issue. The Royal Commission on Health Services, also known as the Hall Commission, was set up to investigate the matter. The CMA believed that the people outside of the "socialist province" of Saskatchewan would be more willing to accept a compromise that was in alignment with the CMA.[23]

Chief Justice Emmett Hall was appointed by the PC government to lead the Commission. After interviewing many Canadians, Hall was surprised by the inequality in access to health services. A few years later, in 1964, to the surprise of many, the Hall Commission's report was strongly in favour of a universal health insurance plan. Hall even went as far as to say: "The only thing more expensive than good healthcare is no health care."[24]

The Hall Commission was highly influential in the creation of Medicare, and it stressed the importance of dental care.[25] The authors of the report expressed concerns about an acute shortage of dentists, who would be unable to meet the demand if the entire population received dental insurance. As such, they recommended the government immediately provide dental coverage to children, expectant mothers and recipients of public assistance.[26] The report also recommended opening more dental schools to help alleviate the shortage in the dental workforce so that dental care could eventually be incorporated in Medicare.

While the CMA stuck to lobbying the federal government, the physicians of Saskatchewan took a more aggressive approach to try to sway public opinion. Many doctors used their status in their communities to misinform the public. Colleen Fuller explains in *Caring for Profit*: "In the eyes of many patients, doctors had a saint-like status — selfless and hardworking, caring for and healing the most vulnerable.

Doctors, therefore, were the perfect moral front for a business sector suffering from low levels of public esteem."[27]

The doctors and their allies in the business community spent more money on propaganda than any political party spent in the 1960 election, even using outright lies to further their cause. For example, they claimed that the state would institute compulsory abortions and could commit people to mental hospitals.[28] The doctors' campaign against Medicare was not effective at stopping the CCF from winning a majority in the legislature, but the doctors continued their opposition to the democratic mandate. When the CCF, now led by Woodrow Lloyd, went ahead with a government-funded universal health insurance plan, approximately 90 percent of doctors in the province went on strike.

The strike lasted for 23 days, from July 1–23, 1962. Doctors, along with local news outlets, business leaders and religious figures, went to war opposing Medicare, with no hesitation towards employing racial slurs, red-baiting and even threats of violence. A few physicians from the United Kingdom who were sympathetic of the fight for Medicare came to Canada to help fill the gap in medical services. Due to dedication and a well-organized base of support by the CCF, unions and activists and the help of a few sympathetic doctors working in community clinics, public opinion for universal healthcare remained high and the striking doctors caved.[29]

The Saskatoon Agreement was signed by the provincial government and representatives of the medical profession, and it had important concessions from each side. The government decided to fund a health insurance plan that permitted physicians to continue working in private practice using a fee-for-service model, and the physicians agreed to cooperate with the government in implementing universal public financing of their services.[30]

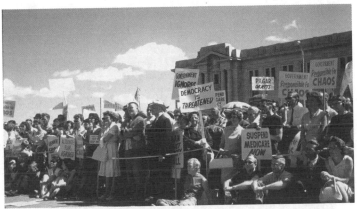

Keep our doctors meeting outside the Legislative Building (Provincial Archives of Saskatchewan Photographic Service Series, R-A12109).

Up until this point, the business community was vehemently opposed to Medicare as it took away an opportunity for them to make a profit from healthcare and they were worried the ideology that led to nationalization, or removing profits from an industry, could spread to other areas of the economy.[31] Politicians in the dominant political parties outside of Saskatchewan either opposed the idea or supported it in rhetoric only. However, due to the popularity of Saskatchewan's universal healthcare plan, the tides began to turn.[32]

In 1961, the CCF came together with the Canadian Labour Congress to form the New Democratic Party (NDP), which was viewed as the champion of universal healthcare.[33] Conservative and Liberal politicians, along with business leaders, worried that the NDP stance on Medicare could result in increased support for the party and even that the NDP could form government either federally or provincially.[34]

By 1966 each province had implemented a universal health insurance plan with financial support from the federal government. The

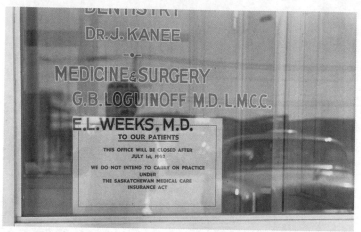

A doctors' office closing during the 1962 strike (Provincial Archives of Saskatchewan Photographic Service Series, R-PS62-229-10).

cost-sharing agreement between the federal and provincial governments was achieved during a federal minority parliament when Lester Pearson's Liberal Party required the support of Tommy Douglas's NDP to govern.[35]

The fight for universal healthcare focused on physician services, with the intention to expand the program to include dental care and other services later. Clearly, that never happened. How did dentists view the prospect of including dental care in the universal healthcare system, and how did they influence the conversation?

The registrar of the Manitoba Dental Association, Dr. W.G. Campbell, echoing the concern of many dentists, declared that the profession would mount militant opposition if the government planned to include dental care in Medicare.[36] Dentists had many of the same concerns that physicians did, which centred on control of the profession and finances, not public health.

Dentists, individually and through their federal and provincial associations, influenced the public and politicians. They argued that including dental care in the health insurance plan was unnecessary and, later, escalating their opposition, not feasible. Their first argument framed oral health as a personal responsibility:

> It's time to tell the public — loudly and clearly — that responsibility for oral health doesn't rest solely with dentists and auxiliaries, the availability or non-availability of the dental team, the number of dentists per capita or even, whether fees are high or low. Just as the federal government is now starting to emphasize its new perspective on health care and the responsibility of the public for many of its own diseases, so organized dentistry must put more of the onus for the dental health of the nation right where it belongs — on the individual.[37]

While individual responsibility is one component of maintaining oral health, it is not the only one. Access to dental care is another essential component, as it helps prevent dental disease and allows the disease that does occur to be treated early on, preventing many downstream problems. The ideology pushed by the dental profession, where the government is minimally involved in funding dental care, would decrease access to dental care and education on oral hygiene and diet, worsening the oral health of society.

Dentists' second argument against including dental care in Medicare was that there was a shortage of dentists. It is true that Canada had a shortage of dentists, particularly in rural communities. A 1939 report commissioned by the federal government and performed by the National Committee for Mental Hygiene highlighted the shortage and distribution of dentists in the country. It stated that the number of dentists required for all Canadians to access adequate dental services would have to grow from 4,039 to 10,362.[38] The report noted that distribution of healthcare workers, including dentists, was determined by the ability to make a living rather than based on people's need for health care. These trends held true in the coming decades as well.[39]

The shortage of dentists had decreased by training more dentists following World War I; many returning soldiers wanted to pursue a career in dentistry and schools expanded the number of students they accepted. In a few years, the number of dentists in the country increased greatly.[40] After the implementation of Medicare, the federal government helped establish four more dental schools.[41] Further, different dental care delivery models require fewer dentists to meet population demand as other members of the dental team are relied on more heavily.

In the context of a shortage of dental practitioners, organized dentistry emphasized that, if governments were to implement some sort of dental plan, resources be focused on children:

> If we are to have a national health program, and every sign points that way, we should emphasize dental care for the child rather than for the adult.... We should urge that, wherever possible, it be done under the system of private practice; we should battle against a lowering of professional standards and the development of a stifling bureaucracy. We all recognize that professional tradition and the ideology of the professional man makes it difficult for him to accept the principle of collective bargaining.[42]

For many, this logic made sense. If there are too few dentists, the moral thing to do was to help the children first. Ignoring the fact that a universal system could place a greater focus on treating children, the dentists' narrative resonated with politicians, and this assessment is what ended up being implemented by governments in the subsequent decades. Even where organized dentistry spoke of a government-funded dental plan for children, they continued to endorse fee-for-service, dentist-centred private practice, which is the model that future governments took when building targeted dental programs.

Concerns about lowering professional standards were common among dentists. They argued that a universal dental plan would pay dentists so little that they would be required to do far more dental work to maintain their income and this would result in lower quality.[43] One only has to look to physicians in Canada to dispel the notion that working in a country with universal healthcare lowers one's income or the quality of care.[44]

The third argument made by dentists was that, with sufficient preventative measures, a universal dental plan would not be justified:

Let it be stated emphatically that organized dentistry is not supporting legislation to merely set up large scale systems of treatment but is proposing a definite plan of approach towards the controlling of dental disease in Canada. The former is retrograde for dentistry, the latter is advance. The [first] means making dentists excavators and fillers of teeth; the other places dentistry in the scientific and professional health category.[45]

The argument was that implementing a universal dental plan would neglect preventative measures and lead to inefficiencies, with dental professionals having to focus on fixing problems rather than preventing them. Considering the inequities that exist in the current private dental care system, there is a stronger argument that these outcomes are a product of a private rather than public dental system.[46]

In the years following World War II, the idea of prevention in dentistry was intimately tied in with a growing body of evidence of the benefits of community water fluoridation (CWF) to oral health. CWF was shown to be safe and reduce the rate of dental decay in the population by 25–30 percent.[47] It was also shown to be cost effective, as every dollar spent on CWF resulted in more than 20 dollars saved in treating dental decay. While CWF does reduce dental decay, its benefits were greatly exaggerated, for example, in this *New York Times* headline: "End of most tooth decay predicted for near future."[48]

Dentists exploited the belief that CWF would end most tooth decay to argue that a universal dental plan would be wasteful and expensive, as it would focus on treatment, whereas CWF would much more cheaply prevent dental decay.[49] These issues are not mutually exclusive; there could be CWF and a universal dental plan. In fact, the reduced dental decay from CWF could have helped alleviate the shortage in the dental workforce and made a universal dental plan more feasible.

Both physicians and dentists were against the idea of universal healthcare. Both had concerns about losing autonomy over the profession and lowering the incomes and standards within the profession. Both professions focused on the perceived downsides of universal healthcare rather than the potential benefits. The difference: dentists won their fight, while doctors did not. Many politicians believed dentists' assertion that a universal dental plan was neither feasible nor necessary and that oral health was a personal responsibility. With activists and left-leaning politicians focusing their effort

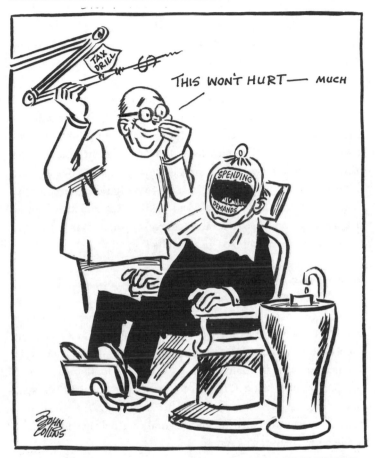

Courtesy of artist, John Collins, The Gazette, about 1964, M965.199.2851, McCord Stewart Museum.

on universal coverage of physician services, there was not enough pushback promoting the narrative that dental care was no different than other forms of healthcare, and the window of opportunity for fundamental change in dental care closed. Soon after Medicare was implemented, federal and provincial governments considered that they were spending too much on healthcare and were keen to keep the cost for services like dental care on individuals.[50]

As a result, provincial governments opted for a targeted rather than universal approach to public dental spending. This meant that public spending focused on specific populations (e.g., children, social assistance recipients) and left most of the population to access care privately. These targeted programs left many gaps in coverage and followed the dental profession's desire to design programs around dentists working on a fee-for-service basis in private practice. Despite this, a bold school-based dental program in Saskatchewan challenged the status quo and achieved great results.

SASKATCHEWAN DENTAL PLAN: THE THREAT OF A GOOD EXAMPLE

In 1962, the CCF of Saskatchewan was on a mission to implement a universal health insurance system that would cover everything, from head to toe. At this time, the CCF government was involved in a heated battle with physicians regarding the implementation of Medicare, which made it difficult to push for other initiatives, such as coverage for prescription drugs and dental care.[51] Nevertheless, the government decided to study dental care delivery in order to implement a plan at a later date.

The CCF identified two main barriers to accessing dental care in Saskatchewan. First, dental care was expensive and thus inaccessible to much of the population. Additionally, many people in Saskatchewan lived in remote locations, and few dentists were willing to set up a practice in these areas.[52] The government looked to methods of dental care delivery in other countries for guidance.

Of particular interest was the New Zealand dental program, which had been providing quality dental care to school-aged children at a modest price for taxpayers for about 30 years. The CCF government sent a group to New Zealand to study the program, which was able to keep costs low by operating out of clinics set up in schools and by employing dental therapists, also known as dental nurses.[53]

Dental therapists differ from dental hygienists in that their scope of practice extends beyond preventative services to include fillings, simple extractions and stainless-steel crowns. The relationship of a dental therapist to a dentist is much like that of a nurse practitioner to a physician. The use of dental therapists proved to have considerable advantages. For one, with dental therapists performing basic dental services, dentists were able to focus their time on more complicated procedures, such as root canals. Additionally, dental therapists' salaries were modest compared to the earnings of dentists, making them a more cost-effective option.[54] With the information obtained from their research, the CCF concluded that the employ of dental therapists was a sound approach to addressing oral health disparities.

Unfortunately, the CCF was preoccupied with its universal health insurance plan and did not implement a dental plan prior to losing the 1964 election to the Liberal Party.[55] Although the Liberal Party, under the leadership of Ross Thatcher, had endorsed school-based dental clinics along with the CCF during the election campaign, nothing was implemented in Thatcher's first term in office.[56]

However, when the Liberals won re-election in 1968, they started the Oxbow Project, which hired one dentist, two dental therapists and three assistants who travelled in a mobile clinic to provide care for children in schools in Oxbow, Saskatchewan. The project demonstrated that dental therapists did high quality work and increased access to dental care.[57] Despite growing evidence supporting the use of dental therapists, major obstacles prevented them from establishing a more prominent role in dental care delivery.

A survey of dentists in Saskatchewan at this time found that a strong majority believed there was an extreme shortage of dentists in rural parts of the province. But dentists opposed the use of dental therapists in school-based dental clinics and favoured a dentist-centred fee-for-service program for low-income children that would be run out of private-practice dental clinics.[58] The powerful dental associations lobbied governments according to their members' desires.

In 1971, Allen Blakeney's NDP came to power in Saskatchewan with a mandate to establish a dental therapy training school and dental clinics in schools across the province.[59] The idea of using dental therapists to increase access to dental care was popular amongst the public as dentists were only serving a relatively small segment of the population. The NDP's minister of health, Walter Smishek, referred to the public's concerns of dentists raising their fees 15–20 percent in one year; Smishek believed dentists had monopoly-like conditions and that dental therapy would be crucial in combatting this situation.[60]

Before the dental plan could get started, the NDP had to create a training program for dental therapists. One training program was run out of the Regina General Hospital and the second was set up by the federal government in Prince Albert, which was relocated in 1981 to Fort Smith, Northwest Territories. Free tuition was offered to attract students from northern communities in the hopes they would return there afterwards to practise.[61] While dental therapy students were being trained, dental clinics were being set up in schools. In 1974, when the first class of dental therapists graduated, the NDP government started hiring them on a salaried basis to work in these clinics. This became known as the Saskatchewan Dental Plan (SDP).[62]

In the first year of the SDP, dental therapists treated 13,070 children, and 37,032 were treated the year after. The shorter time to train a dental therapist compared to a dentist, which was 28 months versus 7 years, allowed the SDP to expand rapidly. The program grew as new dental therapists graduated, to a peak of around 90 percent of school-aged children (166,634) being enrolled.[63]

The rapidly growing SDP was widely popular among parents as it was free at the point of access, and they did not have to arrange appointments at private clinics. School dental clinics meant no lost time from work going to and from the nearest dental office, which for many families, particularly those living in rural communities, was far away. Children were more accepting of school-based dental clinics as they were in a familiar atmosphere. As such, having dental therapists work in schools removed significant barriers to accessing care.[64]

In 1975, after the first year of the SDP, a clinical service evaluation of the dental work in the SDP was completed. The evaluation was done by three dentists who reviewed the dental work done for 410 children, 300 treated by dental therapists and 110 by dentists. The reviewing dentists did not know who did the work at the time of evaluation. They concluded that dental therapists placed fillings that were on average better than those placed by dentists, and that the stainless-steel crowns were of equal quality.[65] The results were indisputable: dental therapists were performing high quality dental work in the SDP. Due to the focus on prevention and early intervention in the SDP, over the first decade of the program, children on average had half as many teeth extracted and 25 percent less dental decay.[66]

The cost savings for the SDP to use dental therapists, who were paid a salary, rather than dentists, who were paid by fees for services, were considerable. For instance, in 1976, the salary of a dental therapist was on average one-third of the income of a dentist.[67] As the program

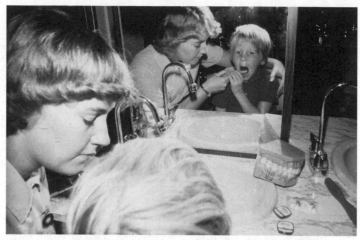

An SDP dental therapist shows a child the plaque build-up on their teeth with a disclosing solution and how to clean it off. "She gives him a pill that colours the bugs red. Now that Glen can see the bugs, it's easier for him to brush them off." Courtesy of Leslie Topola.

grew, the cost per child decreased. In 1974, the first year of the SDP cost the province an average of $341.89 per child, but this figure had plummeted 271 percent, to $91.98 per child, by 1986.[68] In contrast, the private practice–based children's dental plan in Quebec cost more per capita while having a lower utilization rate.[69] In other words, the use of dental therapists in the SDP was a success.

Economist Stephanie Rezansoff explains that traditional fee-for-service private practice dentists did not treat large segments of the population:

> A relatively small proportion of the population is receiving dental care, and … much of this care is received by those in higher socio-economic groups.… The results of this study

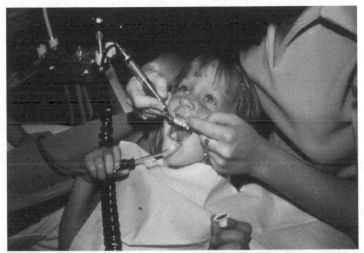

A child having their teeth cleaned by a dental therapist in a school-based dental clinic in Saskatchewan. "Here is the tool that removes the bugs. It sounds like an airplane and washes the bugs from your teeth." Courtesy of Leslie Topola.

[on the SDP] tend to support the contention that changes in the nature of the dental care delivery system are such that inequalities in the receipt of care are eliminated.[70]

The rise of use of dental therapists and the SDP came with opposition, which Minister Smishek noted: "I do not know to what lengths some members of the [Dental] College are prepared to try and sabotage the dental plan even before it gets off the ground." Although the College of Dental Surgeons of Saskatchewan (CDSS) was pushing misinformation about the safety of using dental therapists, it was disorganized and failed to mobilize the public in a way that hindered the establishment of the program.[71]

Dentists continued their opposition to dental therapists and the SDP even as the evidence of the SDP's success was mounting. They were scared that if the public knew how successful this experiment was, they would want dental care for adults delivered in this way.[72] In other words, it was the threat of a good example. The CDSS claimed that dental therapists did poor quality work and threatened that dentists would leave the province in large numbers if the government did not stop using them. Dentists used their powerful, well-respected position and privilege to lobby the government directly for the changes they wanted, which was to privatize the SDP to focus on dentists in private practice.[73]

One dentist who was sympathetic to dental therapists in the SDP wrote an op-ed in the *Moose Jaw Times-Herald* criticizing colleagues: "One must wonder if these individuals place a higher priority on maintaining their monopolistic control of dental services than the dental health of the people of Saskatchewan."[74] This dentist saw the opposition to dental therapists from the CDSS for what it was, a turf war.

The NDP research administrator, Dr. David Penman, expressed frustration with the dental profession: "Meanwhile, the Saskatchewan Dental Association had over many years not only failed to put its dental action where its mouth was; but historically they discussed children's dentistry and its prevention aspect ad infinitum ad nauseum."[75] For years Dr. Penman listened to organized dentistry's concerns for the oral health of children, but he was disappointed that these concerns did not turn into support for actions that would actually improve the oral health of children in the province.[76]

In 1982, the Progressive Conservatives won the election in Saskatchewan. The CDSS, now with the backing of the Canadian Dental Association, saw this as an opportunity to lobby for outright privatization of the SDP. The CDSS wanted to reshape the SDP to replace salaried dental therapists in school-based clinics with fee-for-service dentists working in private practice.[77] At first, privatization occurred slowly by limiting the ages covered by the SDP (ages 5–13 rather than 4–17), but after the Saskatchewan PCs were re-elected in 1986, the privatization ramped up, in part because the party had created a far higher budget deficit than they had disclosed in their campaign. The PCs used the "need" to get the deficit under control as an opportunity to cut social programs.[78]

The PCs took the advice of the CDSS and reshaped the SDP to have dentists working on a fee-for-service basis in private practice clinics. The government claimed that there would be significant cost savings by shifting from school-based dental clinics to private practice, but the shift saved the PCs less than 10 percent of what they had claimed.[79] Worse, the number of children who were seen plummeted. The convenience of school-based clinics in the SDP resulted in 90 percent of school-aged children using the program, whereas children's dental plans in other provinces, which relied on dentists in private practices, had only 45 percent of eligible children using the programs.[80] Privatization of the SDP resulted in 400 staff being fired and 578 school and community dental clinics being closed. Nothing was set up to ensure dentists would locate to the communities where school clinics were shut down, leaving many without access to a dental provider.[81] Within a year, the dental therapy training program in Regina was closed.[82] A similar dismantling of school-based dental clinics also occurred in Manitoba.

The news of the privatization of the SDP came in the 1987 budget, without discussions in the legislature or the public.[83] There was backlash from dozens of communities whose children would no longer receive dental care and debate in the legislature was heated. NDP MLA Douglas Anguish stated:

> This is a very sad day for Saskatchewan families, because
> it marks the official end of the best children's dental plan
> in North America and a replacement of that plan with the
> government's privatized inferior version.... Mr. Minister,
> isn't it a fact that you're in a real hurry to sell off [dental]
> equipment because you want to make it more difficult for
> the next Government of Saskatchewan to reintroduce a
> school-based dental program?[84]

Two years later, a provincial auditor's report showed that $2 million worth of dental equipment from the school-based clinics could not be found or accounted for. The speculation was that the PC government sold off the dental equipment to make it more difficult for future governments to be able to reinstate the program.[85]

The PCs defended the privatization using the same misinformation tactics as the CDSS. PC MLAs talked about dental therapists doing lower quality work than dentists. They also continued claiming that privatizing the SDP saved more than 10 times what it actually did, without mentioning the added costs shifted onto families. The PCs even used the successes of the SDP as a justification for privatization: children had so few cavities that the SDP was unnecessary.[86]

By 2000, children's teeth in Saskatchewan were in bad shape again. A study released that year screened the teeth of 36,000 children in the province and found that 53 percent of six-year-old children had untreated active cavities. This was in stark contrast with the tenure of the SDP, which over its short run greatly cut the need for extractions and reduced cavities and periodontal disease in children.[87]

In 2009, the federal Conservative Party closed the National School of Dental Therapy in Fort Smith, Northwest Territories, which was the only dental therapy training program left in the country. With no training programs, the number of dental therapists in Canada has decreased through attrition.[88] This has a negative effect on access to oral healthcare for children and rural communities relying on dental therapists as few dentists are willing to work in those communities. The Children's Dental Program in the Yukon has already scaled back as there are no longer dental therapists to recruit.[89] In the fall of 2023, a new dental therapy training program will be opening in Saskatchewan.[90] While this is good news, its small scale won't even bring dental therapy back to its previous level of prominence in the 1980s, when there were three training programs, and even then, the field was fairly obscure outside of Saskatchewan, Manitoba and some Indigenous communities.

The SDP was the largest experiment with dental therapists in Canadian history. It challenged the dentist-centred private practice model and showed a way to deliver dental care in a more equitable and cost-efficient manner. Organized dentistry opposed dental therapy because it was so successful. The public-delivery dental therapy model allows for improving public health, but it requires overcoming powerful business interests that benefit from the status quo.

Despite the dental profession's bluster for dental public health, particularly for children, they have opposed crucial changes that would improve the population's oral health. It is clear that these fights have more to do with financial interests and control over the profession than with public health. Since the dental profession has largely gotten their way, where access to dental care is not a right, the government plays a very small role in the funding and delivery of dental care, and dentists face little to no competition from dental therapy, the dental profession has paved the way for the problems we face today. Charting a course that is independent of the dental profession is needed in order to prioritize dental public health over the profession's narrow self-interest.

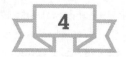

PUBLIC DENTAL PROGRAMS

With dental care excluded from Medicare, provinces have opted for targeted rather than universal approaches to public dental spending. Targeted programs provide resources for care to vulnerable populations, leaving the remainder of the population to access care on the private market. With robust targeted dental programs, most people who are unable to access care privately could receive assistance; unfortunately, the current underfunded piecemeal approach leaves gaps in coverage.

Targeted dental programs were formed in the years after Medicare was implemented. The populations covered by public dental programs largely followed the report of the Hall Commission, which, because of an acute shortage of dentists in the country, had recommended that public dental coverage be extended first to children, expectant mothers and public assistance recipients.[1] Despite the shortage of dentists being alleviated by opening new dental schools in the years after Medicare was formed, the initial recommendations of the Hall Commission are still all that has been implemented.

These targeted dental programs were a response to large unmet dental needs in the population that were deemed socially unacceptable. For example, children were considered unable to care for themselves and therefore worthy of public dental coverage.[2] This paternalistic approach cemented public dental spending as welfare rather than healthcare.[3] The idea of worthiness to receive public dental coverage allowed governments to restrict access when their agenda was to reduce social spending. The idea of worthiness allowed the restriction of both who was covered and what was covered.[4] Many targeted programs only offer coverage for pain relief, and they neglect preventative services and early intervention.

While targeted dental programs are aimed at specific populations, the way these groups are targeted can vary. For example, a program targeting children can cover all children regardless of socioeconomic status, like the SDP did, which ensures everyone has the same coverage and effectively removes private plans. A second option covers only uninsured children, which means that every child has some coverage, but the program keeps the discrepancies between the quality of coverage under public and private plans. A third approach is that children's programs can cover families with low incomes or receiving social assistance. This third method, which includes most targeted dental programs in Canada, creates a gap between those who are eligible for public coverage and those who can access care privately.[5]

Almost all targeted programs in Canada rely on dentists in private practice.[6] Government programs pay dentists on a fee-for-service basis for the limited procedures they cover. These fees are well below those recommended in the provincial fee guides, which are what private plans follow.[7] This discrepancy leaves many relying on targeted programs struggling to find a dentist who will accept them or facing greater out-of-pocket expenses.[8]

In 2018, the Canadian Institute for Health Information found that only 5.76 percent of the $15 billion spent on dental care that year came from targeted government programs. Of the public dental spending, 63.5 percent came from federal programs, 34.9 percent from provincial programs and the remaining 1.6 percent from municipal programs.[9] Some provincial programs are administered by municipalities, which fund a small portion of the program.[10] The 2022 federal budget earmarked $300 million for a children's dental program, which will increase the share of public dental spending by 1.5 percent.[11] The limited scope of targeted dental programs reveals why so many people are still unable to access care.

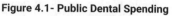
Figure 4.1- Public Dental Spending

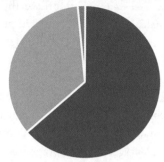

■ Federal   ■ Provincial   ■ Municipal

PROVINCIAL PROGRAMS

There are no federal standards for provincial dental programs, which results in significant variations between jurisdictions in what populations and services are covered.[12] Every province and territory excludes uninsured adults from public dental coverage, though each province and territory provides some level of dental coverage for children and adults on social assistance.[13] Coverage varies across the provinces, from only pain relief to fillings and dentures.

While some programs are better than others, all the provincial programs are wholly inadequate to meet the population's needs. Provincial programs are underfunded and leave large segments of the broader population without dental insurance. The medical and dental

Figure 4.2 Per Capita Public Dental Spending by Province and Territory

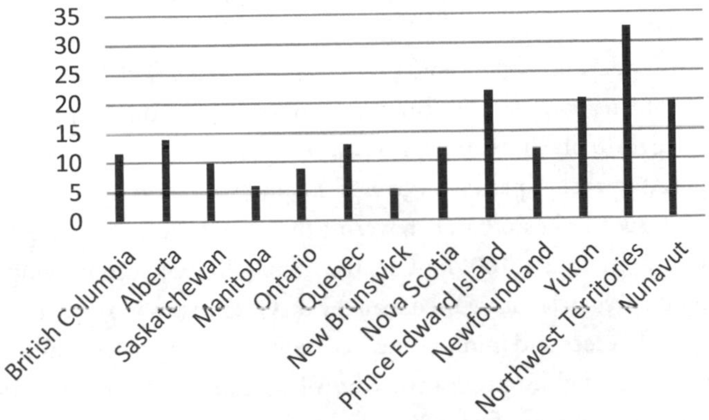

professions, and some politicians, are increasingly acknowledging this.[14] In this section, the provincial programs are broken down into programs for children, adults and seniors, followed by a discussion of dental schools.

Children

While each province and territory has some form of public dental program for children, this coverage varies greatly in eligible ages, income thresholds, services covered and fees. Only four provinces guarantee that children have some form of dental insurance. Prince Edward Island guarantees dental coverage for children 17 and under, Nova Scotia for children 14 and under, Newfoundland for 12 and under, and Quebec for children under 10 years of age. These programs provide dental coverage to the uninsured in the age range, which leaves other children to be covered under their parents' private plan. These provincial plans are beneficial in comparison to the programs only for low-income children or social assistance recipients, as every child in an age range has some level of dental insurance, but problems still exist.

The underfunded targeted programs pay out fees well below what private plans pay, often leaving the families relying on the program to struggle to find a dentist who will accept them.[15] Dentists are not required to accept patients covered by public programs, and many dentists see the fees as barely covering their overhead costs.[16] In 2018 in Quebec, about 1,400 dentists threatened to leave the provincial program, Régie de l'assurance maladie du Québec (RAMQ), in protest over the low fees and minimal services covered.[17] As a result, children who rely on public programs, who often come from low income families that already face a greater burden of dental disease, often access care later, when dental disease has progressed.

British Columbia, Alberta, Saskatchewan, Manitoba, Ontario and New Brunswick have no public dental plans for the uninsured of any age group.[18] All the public dental programs in these provinces are targeted to those with either a low income or on social assistance. For example, Ontario has a program for low-income children under 17 called Healthy Smiles Ontario.[19] British Columbia has a program for children on social assistance and in low-income families that sets hard limits on what it will pay out, which is up to $2,000 every two years, with an additional $1,000 available if general anesthesia is needed in the hospital setting. Costs above this must be paid out of pocket, even if done in a hospital. Structuring programs this way results in greater gaps in access between those who are eligible for targeted programs and those who can access care privately.

The dental departments at children's hospitals are also part of the publicly funded dental infrastructure. This is where children who need general anesthesia seek treatment. Children may be seen here because of their complex health needs or because they were unable to access care until the dental decay became too extensive to be treated in an outpatient setting. The departments in these hospitals receive funding through a mix of provincial and federal health spending and often work in partnership with dental schools.[20]

Adults

No province provides dental insurance to all uninsured adults, and targeted dental spending is limited to those on social assistance and those living with a recognized disability. Since dental programs for adults are targeted to relatively small segments of the population, there are no supports for adults who work and do not receive benefits through their employment. Since fewer employers have been providing work-related dental insurance, access to dental care for the adult population has been worsening.[21] Even for adults eligible for a targeted program, accessing dental care is often an uphill battle.

In Ontario, the Ontario Works program covers "specific emergency dental treatments only" for people on social assistance. In 1997, Ontario Works implemented various surveillance techniques like drug tests and fraud hotlines among others to reduce access to the program,[22] demonstrating how the concept of worthiness has been weaponized against people struggling with addictions and single mothers, in order to justify the government's desire to reduce social spending. For the select few who are eligible for the program, the coverage is limited to pain relief, which means extractions.

Nationwide, all dental programs for adults on social assistance are meagre, with the exact structure of these programs varying. For example, some provinces set a hard limit on how much they will pay out in a certain period. Adults who receive disability or income assistance in BC can receive up to $1,000 for dental care over two years.[23] In Newfoundland, social assistance recipients receive coverage for a percentage of extractions and dentures, but there is a limit of $300 every three years for fillings.[24]

In Canada, people with developmental disabilities often face some of the greatest barriers in accessing care. This is due to a combination of factors, including more time or sedation often required for care, reluctance of dentists to do the work due to low fees targeted programs pay out and a lack of education for dentists in treating people with a disability. As a result, many access care at a late stage for emergencies rather than for prevention and early intervention.[25] The programs for adults with disabilities in many provinces are tied to family income and the provinces' restrictive assessment of whether somebody in fact has a disability.[26] The Ontario Disability Support Program website tells people to contact their case worker to see what dental services they may be eligible for.[27] This method shifts the burden of restricting access to care onto case workers.

While some dentists will accept patients with the lower fees paid out by the targeted programs, others require large copayments or payment of the full fee up front. This means that even though public dental programs exist, many relying on them still have difficulties in accessing care.

Seniors

Seniors are particularly vulnerable to losing access to dental care for a few reasons. At retirement, people lose their work-related benefits, like dental insurance, and have to pay for care out of pocket. Mobility issues and cognitive decline can make oral hygiene and going to the dentist more difficult. Despite these issues, provincial governments in Canada have invested very little in dental care for seniors.[28]

No provincial programs for seniors encompass all the uninsured but rather are targeted to those with a low-income or on social assistance, if the province has any programs at all. In fact, British Columbia, Manitoba, Quebec, Nova Scotia and Newfoundland have no programs for seniors,[29] and other provincial programs are so meagre they barely cover any procedures and have low fees, making it very difficult to find a dentist.

In 2019, the Ontario Seniors Dental Care program was created to cover basic dental services for people 65 years of age and older with incomes of $22,000 or less per year ($37,100 for couples). The program requires people to apply for coverage and seek treatment through public health units and partnering health centres.[30] While the use of public health units over private practice is good in theory, in this instance, it is a way for the government to restrict access to the program by only hiring a limited number of dentists for the units. The program has already faced criticism due to the amount of paperwork needed to become eligible and the too few dentists involved in the program, resulting in long waits to receive care. In cases where long waits are not feasible, patients end up having to find the funds to seek care in a private clinic.[31] Members of the health board of Hastings and Prince Edwards Counties, along with a Region of Peel staff report, have also expressed concerns with the program, ranging from long waitlists, lack of comprehensive services and gaps in coverage.[32]

The Ontario Seniors Dental Care program highlights a problem with programs for those with a low-income or on social assistance. To gain coverage under these programs, a person needs to be aware that the program exists, fill out the application, have a stable mailing address and be able to prove income. This process increases the administrative costs of the program and adds barriers that reduce the number of people who use the program. On the other hand, universal programs or children's programs for the uninsured tend to automatically enroll people with no added hoops to jump through.

Dental Schools

While not technically a dental plan, dental schools provide dental care at reduced cost.[33] People without dental plans are often told to go to these dental schools to access care provided by students.[34] In fact, when polled, three out of four dentists believe that governments should fund dental schools so students can treat marginalized populations.[35] This has led to various outreach projects being implemented in dental schools across the country.[36] Some of these outreach programs also receive funding from the federal government.[37]

Reduced-cost care at dental schools has limitations in bridging the gap for those who struggle accessing dental care: reduced cost dental treatment is still not free and requires proximity to a dental school, treatment by students takes more time, and dental schools cannot accept everyone who needs reduced-cost dentistry.

While a variety of provincially funded dental programs exist, none come close to meeting the population needs. There are still plenty of gaps in coverage, and those who are eligible for provincial dental programs still struggle to access care. No provincial government has been willing to invest in its population and start treating dental care like healthcare. Government budgets are a reflection of their priorities, and the oral health of our society's most vulnerable is not being prioritized.

FEDERAL PROGRAMS

Federal spending on dental care can be divided into two categories. In the first, the federal government has a responsibility to provide dental insurance to federal service employees, and coverage for

Figure 4.3 Federal Dental Spending by Agency (000$)

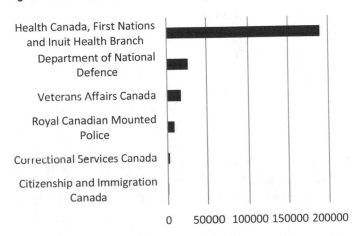

employees of some departments is considered part of federal public dental spending.[38] This category includes members and the families of those who work with the Department of National Defence (DND), Veterans Affairs Canada and the RCMP. These programs function like traditional work-related benefits, although the DND and Veterans Affairs do sometimes directly hire dentists to work in clinics on military bases.[39] The other component of federal dental spending goes towards programs for people in federal prisons, refugees and Indigenous People registered under the Indian Act. These are the programs that are discussed in this section, as they are targeted programs for marginalized populations.

Federal Prisons

The federal government is required to provide dental services to inmates in federal prisons. Correction Services Canada (CSC) states:

CSC contracts the services of dentists and dental assistants, who provide inmates with essential dental care. This
includes fillings, extractions, x-rays and root canals. Inmates
may request a dental appointment, and these requests are
triaged by the dentist. Routine dental hygiene (cleaning or
polishing) is only authorized following an assessment and
diagnosis of dental disease where these services are a necessary component to managing the condition.[40]

While this sounds like reasonable coverage, with federal prisoners being able to get fillings and root canal treatment, the reality is
often much different. A previous president of the Canadian Dental
Association (CDA), Dr. Mitch Taillon, stated to a Senate Committee
hearing on Dental Care in Correctional Facilities:

The majority of services authorized by CSC are emergency
services like tooth extractions and draining infections;
preventive services are only allowed with special authoriza-
tion.… In some cases, dentists who worked in prisons had
their contracts cut from several visits per week to once per
month. As a result, basic preventive services, which could help
reduce the need for emergency care, are rarely provided.[41]

Federal prisoners often receive the bare minimum access to dental
care. CSC does not allocate funds to provide comprehensive dental
care to the inmates, and the agency often has a hard time attracting
dentists from private practice to work in these facilities. Most facilities have no dental hygienists, leaving preventative cleanings as an
afterthought for dentists, who have a hard time keeping up with
emergency and restorative work.

When federal prisoners do not have access to comprehensive dental care, they are often in a difficult situation when their sentence is over. Having missing teeth and visible decay can affect employability, which exacerbates the cycle of poverty.[42] This means prisoners not only face barriers to accessing dental care while in an institution but also once they are released. The consequences of poor oral health are forced upon this population, and if we believe that dental care is healthcare and that everyone deserves access to comprehensive healthcare, then the barriers to accessing that care need to be removed in and out of institutions. This also applies to provincial prisons, where inmates face similar problems in accessing dental care.[43]

Interim Federal Health Program

According to the Government of Canada, the Interim Federal Health Program (IFHP) provides "limited, temporary coverage of health-care benefits for specific groups of people in Canada who don't have provincial, territorial, or private health-care coverage."[44] This program applies to resettled and claimant refugees, recognized asylum seekers, victims of human trafficking and immigration detainees.[45] The length of time a person is eligible for the IFHP varies greatly among the groups listed.

The Government of Canada website states that the dental coverage under the IFHP is "similar to coverage given to social assistance recipients."[46] This means coverage is limited to urgent dental care, which means pain relief. This type of program represents a government acknowledgement of a severe lack of access to dental care for these populations but then doing the absolute bare minimum to help them.[47]

Non-Insured Health Benefits

The Non-Insured Health Benefits program is a federal program for Indigenous People who are registered under the Indian Act (commonly referred to as "status Indians") and Inuk recognized by an Inuit land claim across all age groups. This program does not include Métis and non-status Indigenous People.[48] This federal program helps cover the costs of medical services not included in Medicare, like prescription drugs and dental and vision care.[49]

The federal government states that "NIHB clients do not pay deductibles or co-payments,"[50] but many Indigenous People experience something different. Researchers Ian Mosby and Catherine Carstairs explain: "Many of the Indigenous people who rely on the NIHB Program say that it is often extremely hard just to find a dentist and that, when they are available, dentists often charge additional fees or ask people to pay up front."[51] This is another barrier to accessing dental care.

The NIHB program covers a broad array of procedures, including cleanings, fillings and some root canals and crowns.[52] While this coverage is more comprehensive than many targeted programs, cost savings mechanisms serve to deny coverage for procedures that are nominally covered. The NIHB program uses the predetermination process more than private plans to deter patients from more expensive procedures, which saves the program money. The Assembly of First Nations stated in 2005: "The current system of predetermination for many routine dental procedures causes a prolongation of illness, lacks in compassion and adds considerable cost to the program, particularly if clients have travelled long distances."[53] The use of the predetermination process continues to this day, inconveniencing the people relying on the program and decreasing dentists' acceptance of the program. In some instances, the program has gone to extreme lengths to deny coverage.

For example, the NIHB program has a process of determining whether braces are considered medically necessary. One family, whose dentist believed the daughter would be eligible for coverage for braces under the NIHB program, had to go to court to get the coverage approved.[54] The government spent $110,000 in legal fees to deny coverage for a $6,000 dental procedure. The unpredictability of the predetermination process and difficulty getting claims approved creates significant barriers to accessing comprehensive care.

While the fees paid by the NIHB program are higher than many of the targeted programs, they are still below the provincial fee guides, which private plans use. The fee discrepancy between public and private plans engrains discrimination in access to dental care for populations that have the highest dental needs. The low annual limit the program will pay out also shifts significant costs onto the Indigenous People relying on the program.[55] These factors, along with the increased administrative burden, have resulted in some dentists not accepting NIHB patients.[56] The NIHB program relies on dentists in private practice and does not address the shortage in the dental workforce that exists in many Indigenous communities, leading to an appalling state of access to dental care for many.[57] When speaking on the shortcomings of the NIHB program, Senator Mary Jane McCallum, a dentist and residential school survivor, said: "We've trained people to access care only when they are in pain."[58] Clearly, people with this dental coverage do not have access to comprehensive care.

Federal NDP Dental Plan

There are some signs that these gaps in coverage could soon begin to close. In March 2022, the Liberals and NDP signed a confidence-and-supply agreement that would see the implementation of some

NDP priorities, particularly a dental plan, in exchange for the NDP not triggering an election.[59] In 2019, the NDP proposed a plan to provide dental insurance to uninsured families making $90,000 per year or less, with no copayments for families making less than $70,000 per year.[60] The NDP–Liberal confidence-and-supply agreement states dental coverage will be provided to those under 12 years old in 2022. If the agreement continues, the program will be expanded to cover those under 18, seniors and people with disabilities in 2023, with full implementation of the program by 2025.[61] This program would leave the existing public dental plans in place.

In 2020 the Parliamentary Budget Officer (PBO) estimated the program would cover 6.5 million people and cost $1.5 billion per year once the initial backlog of dental disease is treated.[62] The stepwise implementation of the program will impact the initial spending, as the cost of treating the backlog would be spread out over three years. In 2022, the PBO estimated that the cost of the dental program from 2022–27, which would include the phase-in period and treating the backlog, would be $9 billion.[63] The 2022 budget set aside $300 million for a dental program for those under 12 and $5.3 billion over the next five years. The program will have a budget of $1.7 billion annually once it is fully implemented.[64] The 2022 budget provides funds that are consistent with the PBO estimate for ongoing costs once the program is fully implemented but seems to underestimate the costs of treating the backlog of dental disease.

The Liberals were unable to create an insurance program for children under 12 in time, and as an interim measure are offering cash payments directly to families to pay for dental care until the end of 2023.[65] The NDP have agreed to this as long as a definitive insurance plan is in place by the end of 2023. This is known as the Canada Dental Benefit and will provide two cash payments, one for December 1 to

31, 2022, and can apply retroactively to care received after October 1, 2022. The second payment is for 2023. Each payment will be $650 for each child with a family income below $70,000, $390 for a family income between $70,000 and $79,999, and $260 for a family income between $80,000 and $89,999.[66] This means between $520 and $1300 per child under 12 for dental care from December 1, 2022, to December 31, 2023. By the end of 2023 the insurance program is expected to be up and running for when the program expands to the next stage, assuming the Liberal–NDP deal continues.

As of writing this book, the money has only been set aside for the under 12 years of age portion of the program, which is the smallest of the three phases. The impact of the 2022 portion of the program will be felt differently across the country due to the variation of the existing provincial children's dental plans. Western Canada, Ontario and New Brunswick will see significantly more children covered in 2022 because their existing children's programs only cover either those on social assistance or a low income, where the cut-off is well below $90,000. Uninsured 10–12-year-olds will gain coverage in Quebec, as the RAMQ covers uninsured children under 10 years of age. Prince Edward Island, Nova Scotia and Newfoundland are the only provinces that do not see any changes in coverage in 2022 as their children's programs are for uninsured children up to the ages of 17, 14 and 12, respectively.

It remains to be seen whether the other steps of the dental plan will be implemented, what services will be covered and how the program will influence access to dental care. The effectiveness of the proposed NDP dental program is discussed in the policy discussions section of this chapter and the difficulties with implementation in the conclusion.

Canada Health Act

While routine dental care was excluded from Canada's universal healthcare system, the 1984 Canada Health Act (CHA) does carve out a section for "surgical-dental procedures performed by a dentist in a hospital, where a hospital is required for the proper performance of the procedures."[67] While administering healthcare is provincial jurisdiction, the CHA sets out federal standards that provinces need to meet to be eligible for federal funding. The definition of dental services covered by the Canada Health Act is vague, so it is worthwhile exploring how it has been interpreted.

In-hospital dental services covered by Medicare have tended to be interpreted as specific specialty services.[68] These include surgeries for cleft lip and palate, treatment for oral cancers and pathology lesions, and jaw surgery (whether for jaw fractures or severe malocclusion), among other procedures.[69] These specialty services are covered by all provincial health plans, but the services themselves are often only available in larger cities. For example, residents of Prince Edward Island would need to go to Halifax, Nova Scotia, to access treatment for cleft lip and palate.

While these in-hospital surgical dental services are universally funded by provincial health plans, access to some services remains unequal. For example, in specific instances, individuals with severe obstructive sleep apnea can be treated with jaw surgery, which brings one or both jaws forward to its anatomically correct position and opens up the airway, helping improve the individual's quality of sleep.[70] The jaw surgery itself is performed in a hospital and is therefore covered by Medicare. But the patient requires braces to align their teeth before the surgery, and possibly cavities filled, cleanings and/or teeth removed, none of which are publicly covered. People who cannot afford these additional procedures cannot access corrective jaw surgery, despite the surgery itself being publicly funded.

POLICY DISCUSSIONS

There is broad agreement that access to dental care in Canada is insufficient, but there is disagreement about what to do about it. The debate often boils down to those who believe the existing targeted programs should be expanded and those who argue for a universal dental plan.[71] The current targeted approach to public dental spending is called denticaid, whereas the public funding of dental insurance for all is known as denticare, and it would function much like Medicare.[72] While the denticaid and denticare models differ in the amount of public financing for dental care, they both rely on private clinics. Alternative dental delivery models that rely on public financing of publicly owned clinics also exist. As well, denticaid can take different forms; for example, it can seek to expand existing targeted programs or create new ones, like the Ontario program for low-income seniors.[73] Organized dentistry has tended to focus on pressuring governments to properly fund the existing targeted programs before creating new ones.[74] The benefit of this approach is that it utilizes the existing administrative infrastructure, but a downside is that with so many programs, there will inevitably be gaps in coverage, leaving people without insurance.[75]

These gaps in coverage are what led to the second form of denticaid, where those that are uninsured would be grouped together and given publicly funded dental insurance. This form of denticaid has been the main focus of the Canadian Association of Public Health Dentistry, as it provides everyone with some level of dental coverage and is less expensive for governments and therefore more feasible than denticare.[76]

Denticaid for the uninsured can be implemented in two main ways. In the first, everyone without private insurance would be covered by the denticaid program, effectively erasing the existing targeted programs.[77] Under this model, those currently relying on public plans would see their piecemeal coverage replaced with a comprehensive dental plan. A cost estimate for this kind of denticaid program, which included all necessary procedures, was outlined by Lange, who did the first comprehensive cost comparison of denticaid and denticare.[78] For braces, the IOTN scale, which is used by the National Health Service (NHS) in the United Kingdom, determined whether tooth straightening would be considered cosmetic or medically necessary.[79] While this program is not means tested in that it covers everyone without private insurance, its copayments for adults are means tested. Copayments start at a personal income of $20,000 per year and get progressively higher until they max out at 50 percent for individuals making more than $80,000 per year.[80] This program estimate uses the provincial fee guides, with the cost being $7.5 billion yearly.[81]

In a second approach, denticaid would leave the existing targeted programs in place, and the government would provide insurance to the uninsured. This closely resembles the dental care plan proposed in 2019 by the federal NDP, which would provide dental insurance to the uninsured who have a family income below $70,000 per year, and insurance with a sliding copayment to those with incomes between $70,000 and $90,000.[82] The PBO used the same coverage as the NIHB program for their cost estimate of the NDP plan.[83] While the exact coverage of the NDP dental plan is uncertain, the money set aside in the 2022 budget appears similar to the PBO estimate, so we can assume that the coverage in the new program is similar to the NIHB program.[84] As mentioned, the budget sets aside $1.7 billion per year once the plan is fully implemented and the backlog of disease is treated.[85] If this program actually comes to fruition, it would be the largest investment in oral health in Canadian history and almost triple public dental spending. Even with this being the case, it is worth discussing why the cost estimates for Lange and the NDP denticaid programs are so different.

First, Lange's estimates for denticaid would replace existing targeted programs. If we add the costs of the existing targeted programs into the NDP plan, the total would be $2.7 billion, still far short of Lange's proposal of $7.5 billion.[86] Second, Lange's proposal covers all of the uninsured and all children 12 and under, whereas the NDP plan is means tested.[87] Third, Lange's estimates include comprehensive dental coverage that follows the provincial fee guides, meaning that dentists will not discriminate against these patients.[88] In contrast, the NDP follows the NIHB program and retains the existing targeted programs, which do not have comprehensive coverage and pay lower fees.[89] Since the possibility of discrimination is not present in Lange's program, the cost estimate assumes people would use dental services more as they would be able to easily find dentists willing to provide comprehensive treatment. [90] Lange's estimate also assumes that some employers would have employees seek coverage through the government plan rather than the business providing the benefit.[91]

Having the denticaid program follow the provincial fee guides leads to added spending, but it ensures that those on the public plan are not a lower priority to dentists than those relying on a private plan. Lange's study did not consider that the fee discrepancy between private and public fees could be fixed by regulating the provincial fee guides and placing dental fees somewhere between the existing private and public plans.

Denticaid for the uninsured has benefits over the form that targets specific populations, because the gaps between the various targeted programs are eliminated.[92] Dr. Carlos Quiñonez, a dental public health specialist, points out that the numerous groups (e.g., seniors, working poor, homeless, those living with a disability, the underinsured) having to gain coverage incrementally by expanding targeted programs is not feasible. He states that denticaid for the uninsured may be more difficult politically, but it is "the most expedient way to address existing coverage gaps."[93] In contrast, the Canadian Dental Association (CDA) argues that providing dental insurance to all of the uninsured would be more expensive than the approach that focuses on smaller subgroups and therefore more difficult to get governments on board.[94] Ultimately, the CDA is more concerned with maintaining private dentistry, which is why they focus on getting paid higher fees for the existing programs rather than encouraging greater government involvement overall in dental care.

Regardless of which form of denticaid is chosen, its implementation can be viewed in two ways. First, some form of denticaid is the ultimate goal, and once it is achieved it must be defended. Second, denticaid can be seen as a stepping stone towards the full inclusion of dental care within Canada's universal healthcare system.[95] The NDP MP and health critic Don Davies argues that it will take years to negotiate the terms of denticare with provinces and that the NDP plan could help those most in need while the negotiations occur.[96] Davies refers to the NDP plan as a downpayment on a denticare system.[97]

While moving towards a denticare system is more difficult than staying with the denticaid model, it does not mean that the task should not be undertaken. Lange states:

> There are additional challenges to consider, including dental office staffing levels in rural areas, dentists' operating costs and orthodontic treatments. But none of this should prevent

Canada from committing to a denticare program, which out-performs denticaid in terms of efficiency.[98]

Denticare is more efficient than denticaid for a few reasons. First, denticare is able to spread the risk of high-dental-needs patients amongst the entire population, whereas the population covered by denticaid is higher risk, as they on average have more dental needs, which leaves the more profitable lower risk people in the private sector.[99] Further, denticare would have reduced administrative costs as all claims would be streamlined through a single program, compared to denticaid, which leaves thousands of plans with different rules to be managed (insurance is discussed further in Chapter 5). Denticare would also ensure no gaps in coverage and no discrepancy in fees between public and private plans. This would result in a population with better oral health, which has benefits to individuals and society. The increased efficiency of denticare in comparison to denticaid makes sense as it is similar in the design to the healthcare system. The private US healthcare system, with targeted Medicaid programs, spends almost double the amount of Canada's universal healthcare system, while getting worse results.[100]

Countries that include dental care in their universal healthcare system have been able to put a greater focus on improving public health in comparison to private systems. Japan, a country where 78 percent of dental spending is public, has the 80/20 initiative, which helps people keep at least 20 of their own teeth until the age of 80.[101] On top of ensuring universal access to dental care, the 80/20 initiative supports programs to educate school children and to ensure residents in long-term care facilities receive routine oral care, which reduces the need to treat oral disease.[102] Japan's approach to dental care places greater emphasis on prevention, whereas Canada's approach is to react to disease that has already occurred, which leads to increased spending and worse outcomes. When the 80/20 initiative started in 1989, only 7 percent of Japanese residents who were 80 and older had 20 or more of their own teeth, and by 2016 that number had risen to 51 percent.[103] In Canada, access to dental care has been getting worse, and a person can only keep their teeth into old age if they have the means to do so.[104]

Moving from denticaid to denticare would represent a shift in how dental care is viewed in the broader Canadian society. Historically, maintaining oral health and accessing dental care have been considered a personal rather than collective responsibility.[105] With denticaid, this notion continues to hold, and public dental spending is geared towards those who are collectively deemed worthy of receiving tax-funded care. The number of people considered worthy can vary with denticaid, but with denticare the notion of worthy is extended to the entire population and coverage for dental care would be engrained as a right. Denticare could also seek to integrate dental professionals into the existing provincial and territorial healthcare systems in an effort to ensure people in these institutions receive routine oral care. Helping people brushing their teeth and clean their dentures in hospital and long-term care settings is often overlooked and leads to increased rates of aspiration pneumonia.[106] This acknowledges that maintaining oral health requires some collective action for people who lack dexterity.

Denticare would likely stand the test of time more effectively than denticaid. In order to understand why this is, we have to look at how targeted dental programs in Canada became underfunded in comparison to universal programs like Medicare.[107] Targeted programs have been framed by some politicians and the media as welfare, and they have demonized marginalized people relying on targeted programs as getting "free stuff."[108] This divide-and-conquer strategy fans the flames of resentment of people who are not eligible for free dental care. Cuts to targeted programs are far less likely to engender broad public outrage as the cuts only affect relatively small, marginalized groups.

This strategy has been successful for decades at weakening the welfare state more broadly. Since welfare programs have been effectively demonized, they have been underfunded and weakened. A 2005 research paper for Statistics Canada states:

> Virtually all provinces, with varying degrees of intensity, instituted changes aimed at reducing social assistance dependency. Eligibility rules were tightened (especially for new entrants), benefit levels were cut, "snitch" lines were introduced, and other rule and procedural changes were adopted.[109]

Targeted dental programs have experienced the tightening of eligibility rules, for example, as dental programs for children became programs for children on social assistance, as was the case in British Columbia.[110] The privatization of school-based dental therapy programs in Saskatchewan and Manitoba effectively turned universal programs into targeted programs.[111] This tightening of eligibility inevitably leads to gaps between those who can access care through targeted dental programs and those who can access care on the private market. This is why public dental spending as a share of overall dental spending in Canada has decreased from 20 percent in 1980 to its current 6 percent.[112]

Targeted dental programs have been undermined in other ways as well. One cost-saving technique is de-indexing the fees from inflation, which increases the gaps in fees between public and private plans and further engrains discrimination against public programs.[113] The fees paid out by targeted programs in Canada are around half of what private plans would pay for the same procedures.[114] This results in many dentists not accepting public insurance patients or accepting very few. In a survey of over 1000 dentists in Canada, one in three acknowledged that they made a business decision to reduce the number of patients they see who rely on public insurance.[115]

Many relying on targeted programs have a hard time finding a dentist who will accept them.[116] Even those who find a dentist may worry they will be charged a copayment, or even worse, be required to pay the full fees up front and later be reimbursed some of the fee by the targeted plan.[117] The low fees paid by targeted programs result in higher copayments, which is prohibitive as people relying on targeted programs have low incomes.[118] The experience of a person relying on targeted dental care through income assistance in Nova Scotia highlights this reality:

> Last year I had such extreme jaw pain I landed in the ER. I was given antibiotics and told to go to the dentist. ...When I talked to my case worker, they told me I could get reimbursed for a portion of an emergency appointment, but only severe pain and suffering were considered an emergency. How does one save up to pay the dentist when you don't have enough to buy basic food? Which several weeks are we not supposed to eat to have this money to pay the dentist? How do we wait for a reimbursement? How can we risk the appointment on the chance the dentist determines it's not an emergency (and we won't be reimbursed a portion of the fee)?[119]

Many people believe that those on income assistance get free dental care, but these people often struggle greatly accessing care. Further, targeted dental programs tend to favour extractions rather than saving teeth or preventative care. Underfunding targeted dental programs has also led to certain procedures no longer being covered. Quiñonez states: "Across all programming, emergency services to relieve pain and infection appear to be a universal standard. After that, service coverage is almost completely discretionary. As stated, over time, service limitations and rationing rules have become more stringent."[120]

One particularly cruel way these targeted programs have been cut back is that they no longer cover immediate dentures, i.e., ones that are given to patients at the same time their teeth are extracted.[121] Patients prefer this option because they can have dentures to chew with for the four to six months it takes for the bone and gums to heal after extractions.[122] The base of the denture needs to be remade to fit the healed gums. Because the programs no longer cover that extra step where the base of the denture is remade, people go without dentures for several months, during which time they have great difficulties eating and being social.

For policymakers and politicians, it is worth considering the shortcomings of a denticaid model when deciding whether to expand targeted programs or to work towards a denticare system. Even if the ideal denticaid plan, as outlined by Lange, were implemented, where the fees paid are the same as private plans and there are no gaps in coverage,[123] it is possible the program would be undermined and underfunded in the years after implementation. This can happen through fee discrepancies, delisting certain procedures and tightening of eligibility rules, creating gaps between those with publicly funded insurance and those who can access care privately.[124]

On the other hand, denticare requires buy-in from the society as a whole. When politicians underfund universal programs, they are more likely to see broad backlash in the form of public outrage.[125] This is one reason why funding for Medicare in Canada has increased more or less in line with inflation, whereas targeted dental spending has decreased.[126]

While denticare would improve access to dental care for millions of Canadians and likely stand the test of time more reliably than the denticaid approach, there would still be some problems, and it is worth exploring other models that could do even better. A problem with Medicare is that having insurance does not mean you have access to a provider. Millions of Canadians do not have a family physician, despite everyone having medical insurance.[127] The same can apply for denticare, particularly in rural communities.[128] Without guaranteeing access to a provider, denticare is more likely to react to dental disease rather than being proactive in trying to prevent it.

Public delivery models like the school-based dental clinics in the Saskatchewan Dental Plan (SDP) not only made dental care free at the point of access, but it also sought to guarantee access to a provider. This allowed the SDP to focus on prevention and early intervention in dental diseases, which is why children in Saskatchewan saw large reductions in cavities and gum disease while the program was in place.[129] The SDP was a great example of how to ameliorate the discrepancies in access to dental care regardless of income or geography.[130] The SDP was successful for two main reasons: first was the use of dental therapists, which was a cost-effective way of increasing the dental workforce. Second, that workforce was distributed based on public health needs in easily accessible publicly owned school-based clinics. This allowed dental therapists to be paid a salary rather than the more expensive fee-for-service system.[131] This eliminated the incentive for overtreatment and allowed practitioners to take their time teaching children about how to achieve good oral health through oral hygiene and diet.

The Canadian Centre for Policy Alternatives estimated in 2011 that bringing back the SDP for children aged 5–14 nationwide would cost $560 million, or only 4 percent of dental spending.[132] Considering how successful SDP model was, it is worth applying it to adult populations. Easily accessible, publicly owned clinics could also be set up in high schools, community and Indigenous health centres and along public transit routes, as well as in long-term care settings, shelters and prisons. The efficiencies of applying the SDP model more broadly, focusing on education, prevention and early intervention, would lead to more people keeping their teeth into old age.

In the 1982 Saskatchewan provincial election, the NDP proposed a plan to expand coverage for dental care to everyone by 1986. The plan was to follow the successful model they used in the SDP and apply it to adults. Unfortunately, the NDP lost this election to the Progressive Conservatives, but future governments could bring back this model of delivering dental services.[133]

In the long run, the SDP model is the most cost-effective way of improving the oral health of Canadians. In the short term, there are some difficulties with this model. For one, dental clinics need to be set up rather than using existing infrastructure (e.g., private clinics).[134] It would take time to set up dental therapy training programs and build up the workforce.[135] This model also requires a direct confrontation with the dental profession, but that being said, the denticare and the less bold denticaid approach would also face opposition from the dental profession.[136]

These are the major policy options for Canadians to choose from. denticaid relies on a mix of public and private financing of private clinics. Denticare relies on public financing of private clinics. The SDP model relies on public financing of public clinics. Each of these policy options have benefits and drawbacks in their effectiveness and ease of implementation. Dental public health experts tend to agree that increasing both public financing and public delivery are needed to meet the oral health needs of the population.[137]

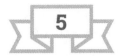

BENEFITING FROM THE STATUS QUO

While Canada's private dental care system has led Canadians to worse oral health outcomes and excessive spending, it has been a boon to some industries. The industries that benefit from the status quo, namely dental corporations and insurance companies, often operate in the shadows, and shining a light on these businesses provides an opportunity to better understand Canada's dental care system.

CORPORATE DENTISTRY

In the last few decades, dentistry in Canada has become increasingly commercialized and has seen an increase in corporate-owned dental clinics. Corporate dentistry is "a growing trend where a dentist (alone, with another dentist or with a non-dentist) owns and operates several dental practices through the use of corporate vehicles."[1] These corporate vehicles, known as dental corporations or dental service organizations (DSOs), have a fiduciary responsibility to maximize profits, the same as any other corporation.

In Canada, corporate dentistry is following in the footsteps of the United States and Australia. Dental corporations are buying up assets of dental offices owned by dentists and taking over control of the administrative aspects of the office (e.g., hiring, firing, bookkeeping). According to Chris Hannay, a reporter with the *Globe and Mail*, "Practitioners who sell to corporate owners typically get back-office support through the firm's technology and staff, help with marketing, and reduced management responsibilities. The buyers, meanwhile, get businesses with steady streams of revenue, and profits that can be boosted by centralizing equipment and administrative functions, and ordering supplies in bulk."[2]

Estimates of how many dentists work in corporate-owned dental clinics are unclear, but industry insiders say the number is growing rapidly and following trends in the US. In 2020 a corporate dental blog stated:

> Canada generally lags behind the USA by about 10-12 years. Looking back at the US dental market 10–12 years ago, a very small percentage of the market was occupied by DSOs. It is very much the same in Canada right now. Currently, about 3 to 4% of the market is occupied by DSOs, whereas in the US it is in the neighborhood of 25%.[3]

More recent estimates from the Canadian Dental Association put corporate ownership of dental clinics with the help of private equity at 6 percent in Canada and 40 percent in the US.[4] This estimate of the corporate dental market in Canada is likely understated. There is a lack of transparency of who owns dental clinics, and the estimates do not take into account different forms of dental corporations, like joint ownership, where the dentist and corporation own the clinic together. The corporation 123Dentist states that a majority of its 350 dental practices in Canada are jointly owned with dentists.[5] Without knowing the true prevalence of corporate dentistry, how can we make an informed view about the consequences of it?

The Dental Corporation of Canada (DCC), the largest dental corporation in the country, advertised on its website that its offices treated more than 2 million people in 2016.[6] In the second quarter of 2021, during the COVID-19 pandemic, the DCC brought in $261 million in revenue.[7] The DCC owns around 500 offices (or 3 percent of Canada's practices), but it does not list its locations on its website, nor do affiliated offices reveal their relationship with the corporation to the public.[8] Hannay states: "In the vast majority of cases, the old branding remains intact after a purchase happens, so patients and customers have no idea their once-independent practice has been taken over by corporate ownership."[9] This is why many people are unaware these dental corporations exist, and it is likely an acknowledgement by the DCC itself that their corporate takeovers would be unpopular and result in the loss of some of their patients.

Despite limited data, experts believe corporate ownership of dental clinics is growing rapidly, particularly among new dentists.[10] Investors in dental corporations are capitalizing on trends in the dental profession. For one, new dentists are graduating with a lot more debt than they used to, often $250,000 or more. New graduates are thus less likely to take out another loan to buy or set up a dental practice, which often costs more than $600,000.[11] This problem is exacerbated by corporate funding driving up the cost of dental clinics.[12] As a result, new dentists are often looking to work for an established clinic with a steady stream of patients so they can pay down their student debts.

Many older dentists are ready to retire and want to sell their dental practice, but with fewer younger dentists willing to buy these practices, a window of opportunity is open for outside investors to buy up dental offices and hire dentists to work in them.[13] Dental practices are attractive to investors because they are profitable; a corporate lawyer working in the field states that they often see a 15 percent yearly return on investment![14] For dental corporations to take advantage of this opportunity, they need to receive sizable investments. For example, in 2018 the DCC received US$900 million from large investment firms to "refinance the Company's existing debt facilities and support its growth agenda."[15] In 2019, 123Dentist raised $425 million in investments with the goal of acquiring 35–45 dental clinics a year.[16] Financing dental clinics this way can lead dentists, who are sometimes personally invested in these corporations, to feel pressured to ensure the clinic brings in enough revenue to pay back the loans and make a profit.[17]

There are several ways for dentists to bring in more revenue. The first is to see more patients who are able to pay the fees, but this is increasingly difficult for a few reasons. For a start, the number of people without dental insurance has been rising as fewer employers are providing this benefit and many people are retiring and losing their work-related insurance.[18] Further, urban areas are often saturated with dentists who are already treating the patients with the means to afford care.[19]

The next option dentists have is to increase revenue from each patient, which has been achieved by shifting the focus in dentistry from routine care to luxury and cosmetic procedures. Some dentists aggressively promote procedures that are not medically necessary, like veneers, implants, tooth straightening, whitening and "replacing old mercury fillings."

The growth of corporate dentistry in the US has exposed how the profit motive can lead to overtreatment and fraud. Considering that industry insiders believe that increasing corporate ownership of dental clinics in Canada is following the trends seen in the US, but 10–15 years behind, it is worth exploring the behaviour of dental corporations in the US.[20] US dental corporations have a history of providing unnecessary treatment and committing fraud. A 2018 report from the American Dental Association states:

> Samson Dental Partners and ImmediaDent were alleged to have engaged in fraudulent billing and excessive and unnecessary treatment. The two companies were allegedly "prioritizing corporate profits over patient care," with non-dentists in management positions exerting influence on dental care decisions, according to the settlement agreement.[21]

These corporations paid $5.1 million in a settlement to the state of Indiana. Alex Pareene, an investigative journalist who studies dental fraud in the US, has referred to a culture in dental corporations where non-dentists encourage dentists to engage in more aggressive clinical decision-making. Pareene stated in an interview with the *New Republic*: "The executive at the top tells the dentists working for them which procedures to push, like a chef tells their team of waiters to push the daily special."[22] Many people expect that recommendations from dentists are standard, but there is a lot of variation. Because dentists and the owners of clinics are paid based on the number of procedures performed, it is understandable that they have an incentive to be more aggressive in recommending treatment, which encourages overtreatment.

In another case, the New York Office of the Attorney General reported:

The state Attorney General's Office has reached a settlement with Aspen Dental Management requiring the company to pay $450,000 in civil penalties and to reform its business and marketing practices after accusing the company of pressuring dentists and dental hygienists at its offices, including six in the Buffalo area, to sell unneeded services to their patients.[23]

According to a US Senate Joint Staff Report on corporate dentistry, Aspen Dental has made similar settlements with three other state attorneys general — in Pennsylvania, Massachusetts and Indiana.[24] Two more dental corporations, Kool Smiles and Small Smiles had to return around US$24 million each after a whistleblower spoke to the US Justice Department about the companies defrauding Medicaid.[25]

Pareene believes that fraud and overtreatment happen more to children: "It intuitively makes sense that there would be a lot of unnecessary treatment and outright fraud on children's dentistry because the evidence will literally all just fall out. You're not going to catch it on an x-ray years later on."[26] There is also a possibility that overtreatment and fraud are detected more often in children due to greater oversight of public dental programs for children, rather than with private insurance. Whatever the case, overtreatment is egregious, and maintaining the status quo allows it to continue.

Clearly, dental corporations in the US have a history of putting profits over the interest of their patients. Considering the lax oversight of dentistry in Canada and the US, it is conceivable that dentists and dental corporations have been pushing the boundaries of what is acceptable without anyone noticing. A person might seek a second opinion if a dentist recommends ten fillings, but would that person do the same if two fillings are recommended and they are required to pay out of pocket for the additional exam? We would expect these concerns of fraud and overtreatment to lead to further investigation and oversight, but it has not, and the institutions that should be doing research into fraud and overtreatment are being influenced by dental corporations.

For instance, Dalhousie University accepted a $1 million donation from the Dental Corporation of Canada, and other dental schools, such as the University of Saskatchewan and the University of Western Ontario, have received similar donations from the DCC.[27] Universities increasingly rely on big money donations rather than public funding.[28] Another such example is the Dental Corporation of Canada donating $250,000 to the dentistry departments of five children's hospitals in the country.[29]

This is a clever public relations move from dental corporations. It allows them to appear charitable while getting a tax write-off for the donations and at the same time influence institutions that are supposed to act in the interest of the public.[30] Dental corporations find access to dental schools and hospitals beneficial, including for recruitment purposes. Further, dental schools may think twice before doing any research into fraud and overtreatment as they risk losing future donations. The charitable donations pale in comparison to the profits that are to be made under the status quo.

Interestingly, at the beginning of the 20th century, organized dentistry had disdain for dental corporations, and dental offices owned by non-dentists were called dental companies. Tracey Adams describes this in *A Dentist and a Gentleman*:

> It was deemed intolerable that licensed dentists would work for laymen. In the eyes of [dental] board members, men could not run a dental company without in some way

interfering with diagnosing dental disease or other aspects of dental practice. Men who employed dentists were considered to be guilty of illegal dental practice. Dental companies were disdained for their inability to allow dentists to practice like gentleman: these dentists were not in a position of authority, but were subordinate to their employers, and they would have to put their employers' profit needs above the needs of the patient.[31]

The dental profession used to be concerned about the influence dental corporations could have on dental providers. Now that dental institutions accept large sums of money from dental corporations and many dentists are personally invested in these corporations, their opinions have changed. Donations from dental corporations are an effective approach to ensuring that dental institutions do not fundamentally oppose corporate, profit-driven dentistry. Dental schools remaining silent on the matter allows dental corporations to continue growing.

Recent years have seen the rise of another type of dental corporation which offers at-home teeth straightening. The most common company doing this is SmileDirectClub (SDC). Customers can either receive a kit to take moulds of their teeth at home or go to an in-store location to get a digital scan of their teeth.[32] The customers' teeth are then assessed by a licensed dentist to decide whether the case will be accepted. SDC claims to only accept mild to moderate cases but when CBC *Marketplace* spoke with an SDC representative, they were told that SDC has an acceptance rate of 97 percent.[33] Taking on cases that should not be treated with clear aligners can put customers at risk of complications and inferior straightening results.

SDC offers clear aligner treatment for around $2500, whereas teeth straightening with clear aligners at an orthodontist's office costs between $5000 and $10,000 CAD.[34] Their lower price allows SDC to market tooth straightening to people who would otherwise find treatment unaffordable. The problem with SDC's business model is that the reduced costs are achieved through providing little to no oversight from a dentist. SDC claims that consumers will be able to speak with the dentist who approved their treatment, but during the CBC *Marketplace* investigation, three out of the four people who were testing the product were told that there was no way to directly connect with their dentist.[35] They were unable to speak by phone with the dentist or receive an in-person exam. This anecdotal evidence is concerning, and further investigation should be conducted. Straightening teeth with clear aligners can lead to complications like receding gums, root resorption, speech issues and cavities.[36] The lack of oversight from a dentist in the SDC makes it possible for these complications to be detected later when irreparable harm may have occurred. SDC defends itself against liability by having patients sign a consent form that states you are required to seek regular dental exams during treatment, where the hope is that the dentist will find these complications. However, SDC makes no attempt to ensure customers see a dentist.[37]

By encroaching on the scope of practice of orthodontists and general dentists, SDC has faced strong opposition from the dental profession and its regulating colleges. SDC argues that "the board has no authority over activities that do not constitute the practice of dentistry."[38] In this case, opposition from organized dentistry is warranted as serious complications can occur with teeth straightening

With this being the case, we must also acknowledge that opposition from organized dentistry to at-home aligner treatment does have an aspect of monopoly control over dental care. While a person should certainly have oversight of their teeth straightening by a licensed dentist, many people cannot afford the $5000–$10,000 necessary to do so. It is no wonder the $2500 at-home aligner treatment is tempting. Dentists have failed to engage with the market of people who want a cheaper option to straighten their teeth; the profession would rather the expensive option be the public's only choice. This has resulted in companies like SDC having a market for their services.

At-home aligner treatment is a natural growth area for corporate dentistry and is likely going to continue to grow. Greenshield was the first insurance company in Canada to begin accepting billing claims from SDC, further legitimizing the at-home tooth straightening business.[39] This partnership is beneficial to both parties. For SDC, if their customers can shift a percentage of the cost onto their insurance, it will lead to more people seeking treatment from them. For insurance companies, it is more profitable if their policyholders use the cheaper SDC rather than traditional orthodontic treatment. This trend further commodifies dentistry and moves the field further from a healthcare service.

As dental clinics become increasingly corporate owned, in whatever form it takes, private profit will be the focus. With greater commercialization, public health gets sidelined. Dentists are spending more of their time doing luxury and cosmetic procedures, which takes time away from medically necessary care. The lack of oversight and research into fraud and overtreatment in dentistry in Canada is concerning and needs to change.

INSURANCE COMPANIES

Insurance companies are one of the main beneficiaries of Canada's dysfunctional dental care system. Private health insurance functions differently than public health insurance, the starkest evidence of which is that private insurance companies have a fiduciary responsibility to their shareholders to maximize profits. To achieve this, insurance companies need to maximize the surplus between the money people/employers pay to them and the amount paid out in benefits.[40]

In their search for ever increasing profits, insurance companies place more resources into finding ways to deny coverage for patients, which leads to insurance companies having significantly higher administrative costs than public alternatives. Estimates have shown that the per capita administrative costs for the private US healthcare system is approximately three times higher than those in Canada's universal healthcare system.[41] This analysis only takes into account the added administrative costs on the insurance end and not the added cost to clinics.[42]

Research has shown that the gap between the premiums paid to insurance companies and the benefits they pay out has been increasing. In 1991, insured group plans for small and medium sized companies in Canada paid out 92 cents in benefits for every dollar in premiums received; by 2011 this number was only 74 cents.[43] While insured group plans for large employers fared better and remained stable over this period, paying out 95 cents in benefits for every dollar in premiums, the set-up of these plans requires some scrutiny.[44] In these large group plans, the employer is assuming the risk by paying the claims itself, whereas the insurance companies are only processing the claims and do not take on any risk. Even with this structure for large employers, the overhead is still double the administrative cost of Canada's universal healthcare system.[45] This is proof that Canadians are not getting good value for their money when it comes to private health insurance.

Insurance companies would rather put money towards initiatives that increase profitability than towards lowering their claimants' out-of-pocket expenses. They increase administrative costs to find ways to deny coverage, and they have marketing budgets, which is why Canadians are inundated with advertisements for health insurance. These techniques occur simultaneously with the risk aversion techniques discussed in Chapter 2, which include but are not limited to copayments, deductibles, yearly limits and prior approvals.[46] These techniques help fund exorbitant CEO salaries and shareholder profits.

It is worth looking at just how profitable Canada's insurance companies are. The following numbers are for the insurance companies as a whole, which includes coverage for things other than dental care (e.g., car and life insurance). From 2011–16, Sunlife Financial made an average yearly profit of $2.1 billion, Manulife Financial $2.6 billion and Great-West Lifeco (now Canada Life Assurance) $3.0 billion.[47] In a public system, these resources would go directly to care.

Despite clearly putting profits over public health, insurance companies still receive favourable taxation rates by governments in Canada. First, all provincial governments in Canada except Quebec provide tax-exempt status for the amount an employer pays towards private health insurance, which creates a $3 billion per year tax revenue deficit.[48] The defence for this tax-break is that it allows more companies to provide dental insurance to their workers. An alternate view is that the tax break is effectively subsidizing the for-profit insurance industry, especially considering that the $3 billion in lost revenue could fund the federal NDP's dental plan for the uninsured two times over.[49] This tax break is even more egregious when we consider that the uninsured tend to pay for dental care with after-tax dollars. In this sense, the poorer uninsured people are subsidizing those who are better off and have insurance.[50]

Insurance companies also use tax haven laws that allow them to legally avoid paying most of their taxes in Canada. One example of this is the Canada-Barbados tax treaty, under which insurance companies that operate in Canada may locate their headquarters in Barbados. This allows insurance companies to shift their profits from Canada to a country where they pay little to no taxes.[51]

Considering how dysfunctional the for-profit insurance companies are to a healthcare system, it is worth exploring why and how they continue to exist. First, the market for private health insurance in Canada depends on how governments seek to address lack of access to care for services originally excluded from Medicare. On one hand, the government can intervene minimally and force people to seek care privately, leaving a large market for private insurance. On the other, the government can expand Medicare by guaranteeing dental insurance for all, which would eliminate the market for private insurance for those services. In between these two options are policies that could eliminate some of the market for private insurance, like a public dental program for all children. This has resulted in the Canadian Life and Health Insurance Association (CLHIA), which is the lobbying arm of the insurance industry, to focus on influencing governments to take a targeted "fill in the gaps" rather than a universal approach.[52] Within the "fill in the gaps" approach, the CLHIA prefers targeting subpopulations (e.g., social assistance recipients) rather than covering all the uninsured, leaving an uninsured population that could become customers for private health insurance in the future.

Since access to dental care only rose to prominence on the national agenda in 2022, it is worth looking at how the insurance and other industries have influenced the discussion on Pharmacare, which has been high on the national agenda for decades.[53] Universal Pharmacare seeks to include coverage for prescription drugs in Medicare, and would reduce pharmaceutical spending by $7.3 billion per year, while ensuring no one avoids their medications due to costs. It is already in place in most countries that have universal healthcare.[54]

The Canadian Federation of Nurses Unions (CFNU) released a crucial report highlighting "big money's three-pronged strategy to stop Pharmacare."[55] The first prong is buying influence through lobbying and advertising. The lobbying of politicians has been shown to increase at times when discussions about Pharmacare are increasing in national prominence. Advertising in traditional media and increasingly on social media seeks to influence public opinion. This is also done by industry groups donating large sums of money to universities and patient advocacy groups. Such advertising and donations have the benefit of creating hesitancy in organizations about pushing for bold changes that would impact their donors' and advertisers' bottom lines out of fear of losing money in the future. Lobbying and advertising seek to moderate the opinion of the public and politicians from bold changes that would lower prescription drugs costs to a more moderate "fill in the gaps" approach, which provides the veneer of progressive change while keeping profits high.

The second prong is to "create an echo-chamber that distorts information and promotes a baseless fear of change."[56] This happens through industry insiders in Canada and abroad funding think tanks, like the Fraser Institute, to write papers that trickle into the media. These think tanks often have a revolving door with people from industries that directly benefit from the ideas being promoted by the think tank. According to the CFNU report: "In 2018 alone, the Fraser Institute published six articles opposing universal single-payer pharmacare and/or supporting Big Pharma-friendly 'fill the gaps.'"[57] Rather than seeing universal Pharmacare as an opportunity to reduce prescription drug costs and ensuring everyone has access to their medications, the narrative can be shifted to claiming that millions of people will lose access to their work-related insurance and the companies will do less drug innovation. These scare tactics seek to protect Big Pharma and insurance companies' profits rather than the public health of Canadians.

The third and final prong is for industry to call for foreign back-up to apply pressure on the Canadian government to protect and preserve industry profits. The industries opposed to Pharmacare in Canada lobbied the Trump administration to put pressure on the Canadian government over a modest reform to control drug prices, which led to the US government downgrading Canada's status as a trading partner.[58] These three tactics, along with donations to political parties, help protect profits of industries that benefit from Canada's universal healthcare system not being truly universal.

Insurance companies and dental corporations in Canada are looking out for their bottom lines, regardless of the consequences to public health. While their profit-seeking tactics have many downsides, some people justify these as necessary to achieve innovation.[59] The idea is that private companies need to be incentivized with profits so they will take the risk of doing research and development. But does this assertion stand up to scrutiny?

The following are examples of public research providing the foundation for modern dentistry. Penicillin, the first known antibiotic, was discovered at a hospital in London, and the technique to mass produce it was developed in laboratories and universities in Canada, all of which were publicly funded.[60] Local anesthetics, the medications that make dental procedures painless, were discovered in a publicly funded medical school in Vienna.[61] Lastly, the development of dental implants goes back to research done by an orthopedic surgeon in publicly funded universities and hospitals.[62] The reasons these bold innovations were made by publicly funded research is because private and public research have fundamentally different priorities. Private companies are concerned with maximizing profits and often see investments in long-term research as risky and unlikely to be profitable.[63] On the other hand, publicly funded universities and hospitals are not subjected to these market forces and can do research that is more long term and foundational. Long-term research is riskier, because if it does not pan out, more resources were put into a dead end. On the other hand, this long-term research can also result in innovations that could not be discovered with only short-term, profit-driven research.[64]

Considering the importance of publicly financed research and the problems that come along with the profit-seeking tactics in the dental field, the next chapter considers how the Canadian government could restructure dental care in Canada to shift the focus from private profits to public health.

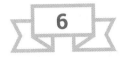

THE FUTURE OF DENTAL
CARE IN CANADA

Canada's dental care system does not have common-sense priorities because the right incentives are not in place. Why does someone who wants veneers get precedence over a child who needs to go to the operating room? Why are dentists busy placing implants while people are in emergency departments seeking relief from dental pain? Why do people vacation in other countries in order get their dental work done cheaper than it would cost at home?[1] These are the consequences of a private system that prioritizes profit over public health. The policies that governments do or do not enact directly shape the priorities of the system. If the policies support the for-profit health insurance industry and dental corporations, then the system will be shaped by institutions that care about their bottom line and not public health.

In Europe, many countries have universal or near universal dental coverage for their population.[2] This is achieved by different policies, with some placing a greater focus on government-funded insurance and others mandating that employers provide insurance and target public funding to specific groups.[3] In Germany the government provides everyone with a base level of dental insurance, but many use private insurance to gain more comprehensive coverage.[4] In many European countries, the private health insurance market is more heavily regulated than it is in Canada in order to curb some of its downsides.[5]

In some instances, rather than a private for-profit company running the insurance plan, it is run by an organization that is mutually owned by the policyholders.[6] This is called mutual insurance, and policyholders can vote on how the plan is run and what is done with excess funds. For example, the surplus could be given back to policyholders directly or used to lower the copayments for the following year.

In the United Kingdom, the dental care that is covered by the National Health Service is effectively a plan for the uninsured. While many people in the UK access dental care through private clinics that do not accept NHS patients, those without private insurance are guaranteed a base level of coverage by the NHS. This coverage is strengthened for certain populations deemed at risk.[7] While years of underfunding and neglect have led to fewer dentists working for the NHS, public spending still accounts for just under half of all dental spending in the UK.[8]

In Denmark, dental care, including orthodontics, is provided to all children under 18 in schools, and there are targeted programs for people with disabilities, the elderly and those relying on social assistance.[9] In New Zealand, dental care for children is provided by dental therapists in school-based dental clinics.[10] In these two countries, dental care for children is included in their universal healthcare systems, along with targeted public investments and subsidies for specific adult populations.

East Asian countries have taken a more comprehensive approach. For example, Taiwan and Japan include dental care in their universal healthcare systems.[11] Japan's system pays 70 percent of the cost of almost all dental services. Many people have private insurance to help with the copayments, and certain populations, like low-income seniors, are given reduced rates of copayment. Japan's dental care system has been very successful at helping people keep their teeth into old age and at decreasing the rate of decayed, missing and filled teeth in children.

While the dental care systems described above are not perfect, particularly after decades of neoliberal-driven austerity, they show that policy options that provide greater equity in access to dental care are achievable. These policies directly shape the priorities of the dental system, with countries that include dental care in their universal healthcare system having more equitable outcomes than those where the private sector is dominant.

THE POLITICS OF CHANGING DENTAL CARE

In terms of moving forward with a more equitable dental policy in Canada, advocates need to know what policies they want and to develop a strategy for how they are going to achieve these policies. The strategy needs to include short- and long-term goals that help gauge progress, and it should focus on placing organized pressure on politicians at both provincial and federal levels to obtain specific policy changes that increase access to dental care.[12] In Canada, universal healthcare was achieved in an incremental manner through a mix of provincial and federal initiatives, and this could also apply to dental care.

On one hand, public pressure could lead a provincial government to championing access to dental care, as Tommy Douglas and the NDP did with Medicare.[13] It took more than a decade to implement universal healthcare in Saskatchewan, starting with insurance for hospital services in 1946. A similar situation would likely be true with universal dental care. It takes time to set up dental therapy training programs and hire graduates to work in publicly owned dental clinics. It would also take time for provincial governments to negotiate a cost-sharing agreement with the federal government.

In 2018 and 2022, the Ontario NDP under the leadership of Andrea Horwath proposed a dental plan that would cover the 4.5 million uninsured people in the province at a cost of $1.2 billion per year.[14] The NDP lost both these elections to the Progressive Conservatives. In order for the NDP to increase its chances of winning in the future, it is important that popular issues like dental care be highlighted during non-election seasons. With 86 percent of the public supporting a dental plan for the uninsured, it seems the NDP has struggled turning their popular proposals into seats in the legislature.[15]

On the other hand, the federal government can take the lead on dental care, and this would most likely take place during a minority parliament where the Liberals are propped up by the NDP.[16] The NDP would have to leverage their support for the Liberals in exchange for public dental spending, although the current political landscape does present more difficulties for the NDP to get concessions. In the 1960s the Pearson Liberals had fewer options to gain support, which helped the Douglas NDP to achieve some of their goals.[17] In the 21st century, the Liberals can potentially seek support from the Bloc Québécois or the Conservatives if they are not willing to meet the NDP demands.[18]

Jagmeet Singh's NDP placed dental care as a high priority when negotiating the confidence-and-supply agreement during the minority parliament with the Trudeau Liberals.[19] On March 22, 2022, the Liberals agreed to implement the NDP dental plan in a stepwise fashion, along with other concessions, in exchange for support from the NDP in votes of confidence until the 2025 election.[20] The dental plan would be for the uninsured with family incomes below $90,000 per year, with a sliding copayment for those with incomes above $70,000. The stepwise implementation plan was to create a program for those under 12 years of age in 2022, expanding it to under 18, seniors and persons living with a disability in 2023, with the remainder of the uninsured people below the income threshold to be included in the program in 2025.[21] If fully implemented, this program is estimated to insure between 7 and 9 million Canadians and cost approximately $1.7 billion per year after the initial backlog of dental disease is treated.[22]

Table 6.1 Proposed Timeline for Implementation of Federal Dental Program

Year	Groups
2022	12 and under
2023	18 and under
	Seniors
	People living with a disability
2025	Remaining uninsured people below income cut-off

Source: Nick Boisvert, "Everything we know about the Liberal-NDP dental care proposal," CBC News (2022). cbc.ca/news/politics/liberal-ndp-dental-plan-1.6393981.

If implemented, this plan would be the largest investment in oral health in Canadian history, almost tripling Canada's public dental spending. The April 2022 federal budget set aside $300 million for the under-12 portion of the program. However, as described in Chapter 4, the Liberals were unable to create an insurance program for children under 12 in time, and as an interim measure are offering cash payments directly to families to pay for dental care. Further, if the confidence-and-supply agreement falls apart before the definitive dental plan is in place, the cash payments could disappear without an insurance plan replacing it.

For the dental plan to come to fruition, the Liberals need to believe the NDP are willing to follow through with their threat to withdraw support if the Liberals fail to keep their promises.[23] The Liberals are aware that polling would influence the NDP's willingness to potentially trigger an election, and they could renege on their commitments if they are polling in a range where they could win a majority government. The NDP may choose not to trigger an election out of fear of moving from a minority to majority Liberal parliament. In another scenario, the NDP could vote against the Liberals in a vote of confidence, but the Bloc Québécois or the Conservatives could vote with the Liberals to avoid an election.[24] Former NDP leader Ed Broadbent has warned that the Liberals may not keep their promises and that the public needs to keep up the pressure to make it more difficult for them to back down.[25]

The NDP dental plan would fill many of the gaps in coverage left from the existing inadequate public programs and the increasing number of low- and middle-income jobs that do not provide dental coverage. The program would also help many seniors who lose coverage when they retire. While the NDP plan is a great start, it should not be viewed as the end goal. With the NDP program, dentists will still prefer to treat people who rely on private plans due to the higher fees paid. Those who are underinsured on the current public programs will still be left with inadequate coverage. Many people will still struggle to afford the out-of-pocket expenses, and plenty of middle-income Canadians will still lack dental insurance. Further, the gravy train will continue for dental corporations and insurance companies. In this context, the NDP dental plan should be seen as a stepping stone to a universal system.

While it appears that the NDP dental plan will be administered federally to speed up its implementation, over time the administrative control may be shifted to provinces through a cost-sharing agreement.[26] Having provinces administer the new dental program from the beginning would slow the start of the program and likely prevent it from being implemented before the next election, in 2025. In the long run, transferring administration of the program to provinces can create an opportunity to establish national standards for dental care in the same way the federal government does with medical care under the Canada Health Act. This means the federal government would place conditions on its funding of the dental program, and if provinces do not meet these standards, they risk losing out on the much-needed transfer payments.

The five principles of the Canada Health Act are as follows:

1. comprehensiveness: all medically necessary services must be covered;
2. accessibility: people must have reasonable access to these services without charge or user fees;
3. portability: access to care is available even outside of home provinces;
4. universality: everyone must be covered for all medically necessary procedures; and
5. public administration: the province must administer the program and be accountable for the funds.

Including the principles of the Canada Health Act as part of the conditions for the transfer payments to the provinces for dental care would be a great start. Other conditions could be added, such as effective regulation of overtreatment, limits on wait times for children needing dental surgery and the setting up of publicly owned clinics in dental deserts, i.e., areas with an insufficient dental workforce. The conditions tied to transfer payments would be an effective approach to creating and upholding national standards for dental care, even when governments that are hostile to the program are in power.

Universal Dentalcare

Clearly, Canada's dental care system is dysfunctional, and Chapter 4 explores policy options that would ameliorate some of these problems, but ultimately, what is the ideal solution? In order to address the core flaws of Canada's dental care system, policy must convert both the funding and delivery of care from the profit-seeking private sector to the health-focused public sector. The public sector has the ability to treat dental disease as a public health problem to be solved, whereas the private sector can only chase profits. This system of public financing and increasingly public delivery of dental care is known as "universal dentalcare," a concept conceived through conversations held in a group I founded in January 2020 called the Coalition for Dentalcare. We are health professionals, students and members of the public who highlight the shortcomings of Canada's dental care system while advocating for a more humane alternative. Universal dentalcare seeks to take the beneficial elements of both denticare and the school-based dental therapy model used in the SDP to create the most efficient system possible.

With denticare, there is public financing of dental care for all, but delivery remains in private practices. Universal dentalcare takes the public financing of dental care for all from the denticare model but prefers delivery to be in publicly owned clinics. This design learns from the strengths of Canada's universal healthcare system while overcoming its weaknesses. A core component of universal healthcare in Canada is that everyone is guaranteed health insurance throughout life, and this is essential to universal dentalcare. This insurance would make dental care free at the point of access, which means there would be no out-of-pocket expenses that could deter people from accessing care. Having the government provide dental insurance to all would provide stability, as people would not have to worry about losing work-related coverage for an essential health service when they retire, become unemployed or lose spousal benefits. If the entire population had quality dental insurance throughout their lives, far greater numbers of people would seek preventative services and early intervention. Oral health outcomes would improve, which has many benefits to the health and well-being of individuals and society.

With everyone relying on the same publicly financed dental plan, dentists would no longer have a preference for treating people who have private plans. This would ensure that those with poorer oral health receive more dental services than those with better oral health. In other words, dental care would be provided based on need rather than ability to pay. Universal programs tend to create a sense of pride in society as everyone relies on the same program, whereas targeted programs create tension between those who are eligible and those who are not. This phenomenon was described by the Swedish social researchers Walter Korpi and Joakim Palme:

> By practicing positive discrimination of the poor, the targeted model creates what amounts to a zero-sum conflict of interests between the poor on the one hand and, on the other, the better-off workers and middle classes, who have to pay for the benefits of the poor without themselves receiving any benefits. The targeted model thus tends to drive a wedge

between the short-term material interests of the poor and
the rest of the population.[27]

Such tensions within the working class are easily exploited to reduce
benefits to the poor, whereas universal programs create a sense of
solidarity in protecting a program that everyone uses. This pride
means universal dentalcare would fundamentally shift public dental
spending from welfare to healthcare and would not be as susceptible
to funding cuts as denticaid. Funding cuts would receive a much
broader backlash if they are seen as an attack on society as a whole.
Considering that everyone would be relying on the program, universal
dentalcare would have to be of high quality to keep everyone happy.

This is beneficial for the public relying on the universal program
but also for dentists. Many dentists fear the expansion to a universal
dental plan will result in them only getting paid the low fees that
currently exist for targeted programs. A universal program would
be funded more reliably than targeted programs and would have to
pay dentists sustainable fees. Further, a universal dental plan would
provide dentists with more patients to treat, benefiting dentists and
patients by allowing people to access comprehensive care. This means
people could save their teeth rather than opting for the cheaper
extractions.

Guaranteeing publicly financed dental insurance would also
encourage dentists to set up clinics in communities where there is a
need for basic dental care as opposed to being deterred by the socioeconomic status of the individuals within the community. Universal
insurance through denticare would help ameliorate some of the
disparities in dentist-per-capita ratios in poor versus affluent communities. While universal insurance would help with this problem,
it would not eliminate it, as seen with Medicare in Canada.

A shortcoming of insurance-based programs is that having insurance does not mean you have access to a provider. This makes insurance-based programs more prone to reacting to dental disease once it has occurred. In comparison, a system that seeks to guarantee access to a dental provider would allow more focus on prevention and early intervention. To address this problem, universal dentalcare would expand the dental workforce, which would include dental therapists, hygienists, assistants, denturists and dentists, among others, and distribute that workforce based on public health needs. The Saskatchewan Dental Plan, discussed in Chapter 3, was a great example of how this could be done. The SDP expanded the dental workforce in a cost-efficient manner by bringing dental therapy into the mainstream. These dental providers worked on a salary in easily accessible school-based clinics. The combination of these two factors led to the virtual elimination of the disparities in access to dental care for children from rich versus poor and urban versus rural communities.

Under a public ownership model, salaried providers could take the time needed to treat people with more complex oral health needs, rather than feeling rushed to get to their next patient like practitioners do under the fee-for-service model. This would be particularly beneficial for disabled people and those who are fearful of the dentist, as the added time would allow providers to find out how to accommodate their specific needs. Having salaried providers also removes the incentive to overdiagnose dental disease, whereas the fee-for-service model encourages it.

Since cost is only one barrier to accessing dental care, publicly owned clinics can be designed in ways that reduce the other barriers, such as accessibility and geography. Having dental care providers work in easily accessible clinics ensures that people not only have dental insurance but also access to a provider. It is much easier to bring a dental therapist to a long-term care facility than it is to have each person in the facility brought to the nearest private clinic. This model should embed dental care providers within the existing provincial and territorial healthcare systems, which would include ensuring patients receive routine oral care when in hospitals and long-term care homes, which is often overlooked and leads to increased cases of aspiration pneumonia as people inhale the bacteria in the plaque buildup on their teeth. This means residents would be more likely to access comprehensive care rather than just pain relief, and a great deal of dental disease could be prevented. Since some publicly owned clinics would be in specialized settings, they could be designed in ways that are more accessible for those populations. For example, clinics in long-term care settings could have added measures to make sure they are wheelchair accessible.

Public ownership is an opportunity to expand the dental workforce to include the use of dental therapists and dental hygienists. Organized dentistry has fought to exclude dental therapy from the mainstream in Canada, and public ownership of dental clinics is an opportunity to change this.[28] Dental therapy would be a cost-efficient way to fill the gap for dental deserts, communities that currently do not have a sufficient dental workforce to meet the populations needs. Many rural communities have little to no dental workforce, and publicly owned clinics could be set up in these communities, with dental therapists, hygienists and denturists doing the bulk of the work. Publicly owned dental clinics like this would work well in schools, long-term care facilities, prisons and community and Indigenous health centres, among other locations. Clinics could be placed next to public transit routes to ensure easy accessibility.

It is important that dental therapists only work in publicly owned clinics. If dental therapists work in private practices, the cost savings from using them would accrue to the owners of the private practice rather than the public. Further, allowing dental therapists to work in private practice would greatly hinder the public sector's ability to recruit them to work in poor and rural communities, which happened in the SDP in the 1980s.

These publicly owned clinics with dental therapists are an essential component of the Coalition for Dentalcare's vision, but universal dentalcare does not need to be in place for these clinics to be built. Governments can start now setting up these clinics to treat underserved populations. If the federal NDP's dental plan comes to fruition, there will be many people who gain coverage but are unable to find a dental provider willing to do comprehensive treatment. The same is true for those who rely on the existing public dental programs. Publicly owned clinics are the perfect place to help these people.

Considering the opposition from organized dentistry to the SDP and the inclusion of dental care in Medicare, it is safe to say there will be strong opposition to universal dentalcare. Building publicly owned clinics with dental therapists in the meantime could create leverage for future governments that want to bring dental care fully under Canada's universal healthcare system. If organized dentistry does not negotiate the terms of a universal system in good faith, then the government can continue building these clinics and bringing dental therapy further into the mainstream until they cooperate. These publicly owned clinics could ensure access to care if private dentists ever went on strike like physicians did during the creation of Medicare.

In order to grow the public dental sector, a dental therapy training program would have to be established. In 2021, a partnership between the Northern Inter-Tribal Health Authority, Saskatchewan

Polytechnic, Northlands College and the University of Saskatchewan received $150,000 from Indigenous Services Canada to develop dental therapy program in Canada. Their proposal was approved, and the first class will begin in the autumn of 2023. While this is a great start, the program will only graduate 21 students per year, which is well below what the population needs.[29]

In the past, dental therapy was a standalone field, but there can also be dual-trained dental hygienists and therapists. This means there could be combination dental therapy and dental hygiene degrees and also programs where dental hygienists could return to school to learn the skills to become a dental therapist. The more than 30,000 dental hygienists in Canada who already have significant dental knowledge are a great asset to grow the workforce and increase access to preventative and restorative care.[30] There can be combinations of these programs across the country, but there would need to be standardization across the different programs.

The dental workforce can also be expanded by reforming how internationally trained dentists come to Canada. Many foreign-trained dentists want to practise in Canada, but the burdensome process for entry acts as a deterrent. Foreign-trained dentists need to take several tests, each of which costs thousands of dollars, before they can apply to Canadian dental schools, which have very few seats set aside for foreign-trained dentists.[31] Two years of schooling cost $150,000.[32] The Canadian government could make it less burdensome for foreign-trained dentists to enter the country in exchange for a commitment to work in underserved communities in publicly owned clinics for a period of time after graduation. The same could be applied to domestic dental students, who also pay absurdly high tuition rates.[33] This is already done for dental students who join the military, and it could be done elsewhere.[34] Generous benefits like pensions and maternity/paternity leave could attract more oral health professionals to the public system.

The interests of both dentists and insurance companies do not align with admitting more foreign-trained dentists or bringing dental therapy into the mainstream. For the dental profession, more foreign-trained dentists and dental therapists would mean increased competition. For insurance companies, more dental providers mean more billing to insurance companies, which decreases profitability. The public ownership model would be a great point of leverage to overcome these hurdles and increase the dental workforce while also benefitting public health.

The public ownership model could also help with the problem of dental corporations. With a dental insurance model of public dental spending and no other reforms, dental corporations would gain access to the public purse. This would lead to a form of public-private partnership that would increase spending without added benefits.[35] In order to create a sustainable public dental care plan, the dental corporations need to be excised from the system. If the right conditions were in place, dental corporations could be nationalized and used as public dental infrastructure that seeks to further public health rather than maximize profits.

Governments could use some of the techniques that dental corporations use, but for the public good. For example, a crown corporation could be set up to buy dental equipment and supplies in bulk, greatly reducing the per unit cost.[36] This is a technique that could entice dentists to work in the universal dentalcare system, even if in private practices. Dentists could gain access to this lower cost equipment and supplies if almost all their work is done within the public system.

While the goal of universal dentalcare is to grow the public dental sector, it is unreasonable to expect that all private practice dental clinics will disappear overnight. At first, governments should focus on building publicly owned clinics to treat underserved communities, and over time the public sector should take over a greater share of the medically necessary dental work for the population. Universal dentalcare needs to find a way to engage private dental clinics while minimizing the downsides of this model. This means that some rules would need to be in place, like regulation of prices and overtreatment/fraud that is independent of the dental profession. With all the dental claims streamlined through a single plan, universal dentalcare would help acquire the data necessary to know which decisions are based on scientific evidence and which on opinion. This will help re-establish trust in the dental profession and shift public opinion towards seeing dentists as healthcare providers rather than as business people.

Historically, public ownership of clinics did not come from the medical profession, and its origins highlight an important lesson in how our society makes decisions. In the years before universal health insurance was implemented in Saskatchewan, community medical clinics (publicly owned) were set up to treat people based on need. Supporters of these clinics were strong advocates of universal healthcare and wanted space for public funding of community clinics within that system. Many believed that public funding of community clinics would promote greater democratic input into how medical care was provided, which would allow for more focus on prevention. This was noted by Stan Rands in *Privilege and Policy*: "Physicians tend to seek medical solutions to social problems. Thus, the clinics (private practices) opened minor surgeries, pharmacies, and optometries, but they did not hire social workers or community developers."[37]

Rands and advocates of community clinics view healthcare as more than just treatment but rather as a holistic system that helps

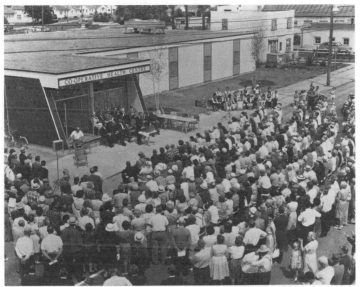

Grand opening of the Prince Albert Co-operative Health Centre in 1964 (Provincial Archives of Saskatchewan Photographic Service Series, S-B8305, photo #13)

people live healthy dignified lives. In the context of dentistry, publicly owned clinics could allow for easy accessibility and a focus on education, prevention and early intervention. Since most dental diseases are preventable, this would be beneficial from both public health and financial points of view. Universal dentalcare should look at metrics like the percentage of people who keep their teeth into old age as a sign of success.

The Saskatchewan NDP were put in a difficult situation when physicians went on strike, and they felt the need to make concessions in order to move forward with the first universal healthcare system in North America. Unfortunately, these concessions meant that the community clinics would no longer be sustainable after signing the Saskatoon Agreement. This ensured that public financing of private clinics would dominate the new system. Rands explains:

> The government of the day consciously chose to avoid further conflict with the organized medical profession and, in doing so, promoted fee for service medicine (private practice) and the continued dominance of the health care system by the medical establishment.[38]

Excluding community clinics from Canada's universal healthcare system was a mistake. It was done to appease the medical profession, which had already been trying to undermine the community clinics long before the Saskatoon Agreement.[39]

When building universal dentalcare, there needs to be a grassroots movement that is strong enough that politicians do not have the leeway to concede to the professions involved. It is time to stop looking to professions for answers to problems in which they clearly have a conflict of interest. This was shown in how the dental profession acted towards the SDP and how both the medical and dental professions treated the idea of universal healthcare. Some self-regulating professions in Canada have used their power to stand in the way of progress rather than helping with the process.

A 2009 poll of Canadian dentists found that only 15 percent believe the government should provide dental insurance to everyone without private coverage, something that 86 percent of the public agrees with.[40] How might the dental profession and other monied interests like the insurance industry and dental corporations respond if a government tries to implement the even bolder universal dentalcare? These interests clearly have an outsized voice in the democratic process, and overcoming this financial voice is necessary to build a better society. It requires a population that is actively engaged with the democratic process, as it is not enough to just show up to the polls every few years.

The movement advocating for universal dentalcare should not shy away from confronting the monied interests that stand in the way of progress. Access to dental care is one of several social components that shape a person's oral and overall health, and these other parts should not be overlooked. These issues include, but are not limited to, income inequality, housing and food insecurity, lack of clean water infrastructure, racism and poverty.[41]

Universal dentalcare is an opportunity to lessen inequality in Canada in two ways. First, everyone deserves to smile, chew and live without dental pain. Currently, a person's smile is a class marker, and universal dentalcare seeks to minimize this problem by ensuring that everyone has access to dental care. Good oral health being a sign of status is also a reflection of wealth inequality in the broader society. How governments pay for universal dentalcare could lessen inequality by shifting the cost of care from regular people under the private system to the incredibly wealthy under a public system. From March 2020 to January 2022, during the COVID-19 pandemic, Canadian billionaires added $111 billion to their wealth while most Canadians were struggling.[42] Universal dentalcare can take a bite out of inequality by shifting the cost of this program onto the wealthy through a wealth tax and cracking down on tax havens.[43]

While the topics discussed throughout this chapter are bold, it is important to remember that they are achievable. The great achievements of our time, such as Medicare, were once viewed as unreasonable. Through hard work, dedication and organization we can shift the political landscape to take power from the wealthy and put it into the hands of regular people. Only by doing this is universal dentalcare possible.

Clearly, oral health and access to dental care are of the utmost importance. The actions currently being made by governments to address lack of access to dental care are wholly inadequate. The history of dental care in Canada shows how we got the flawed system we have in place. People have amassed tremendous wealth and power from the current system, and they will continue to wield that power to maintain the system that has benefitted them at the public's expense. This is why public pressure is essential to building a movement that can confront the core problems in order to implement a system that prioritizes public health over profits. Dental care is healthcare, and it is time the government starts treating it that way.

The Coalition for Dentalcare welcomes anyone interested in building public pressure to change the current dental care system. Please join by emailing us at coalitionfordentalcare@gmail.com.

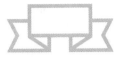

NOTES

Chapter 1: The Struggle for Oral Health

1. Heidi Ledford, "Rot, drills and inequity: The tangled tale of teeth," *Nature*, May 22, 2018. nature.com/articles/d41586-018-05236-4.

2. Bruce Pihlstrom, Bryan S. Michalowicz and Newell W. Johnson, "Periodontal diseases," *Lancet*, 366, 9499 (2005): 1809–1820.

3. Wagner Marcenes, Nicholas Kassebaum, Eduardo Bernabé, Abraham Flaxman, Mohsen Naghavi, Alan Lopez and Christopher Murray, "Global burden of oral conditions in 1990–2010: A systematic analysis," *Journal of Dental Research*, 92, 7 (2013): 592–597.

4. Sato Yuuji, Shogo Minagi, Yasumasa Akagawa and Tooru Nagasawa, "An evaluation of chewing function of completed denture wearers," *Journal of Prosthetic Dentistry*, 62, 1 (1989): 50–53.

5. Centers for Disease Control and Prevention, "Oral health conditions," November 3, 2020. cdc.gov/oralhealth/conditions/index.html.

6. Abeer Khalid and Carlos Quiñonez, "Straight, white teeth as a social prerogative," *Sociology of Health and Illness*, 37, 5 (June 2015): 782–796.

7. See, for example, S. Kershaw, J.T. Newton and D.M. Williams, "The influence of tooth colour on the perceptions of personal characteristics among female dental patients: Comparisons of unmodified, decayed and 'whitened' teeth," *British Dental Journal*, E9 (2008): 204.

8. Vahid Ravaghi, Carlos Quiñonez and Paul J. Allison, "The magnitude of oral health inequalities in Canada: Findings of the Canadian health measures survey," *Community Dentistry and Oral Epidemiology*, 41, 6 (2013): 490–498.

9. Canadian Academy of Health Sciences (CAHS), *Improving Access to Oral Health Care for Vulnerable People Living in Canada* (2014): Fig. 2.2. https://cahs-acss.ca/wp-content/uploads/2015/07/Access_to_Oral_Care_FINAL_REPORT_EN.pdf.

10. Brandy Thompson, Peter Cooney, Herenia Lawrence, Vahid Ravaghi and Carlos Quiñonez, "The potential oral health impact of cost barriers to dental care: Findings from a Canadian population-based study," *BMC Oral Health* 14, 1 (2014): 1–10.

11. Malini Chari, Vahid Ravaghi, Wael Sabbah, Noha Gomaa, Sonica Singhal and Carlos Quiñonez, "Oral health inequality in Canada, the United States and United Kingdom," *PLOS One* (May 2022).

12. David Locker, John Maggirias and Carlos Quiñonez, "Income, dental insurance coverage, and financial barriers to dental care among Canadian adults," *Journal of Public Health Dentistry*, 71, 4 (2011): 327–334.

13. A. Singh, M. Peres and R. Watt, "The relationship between income and oral health: A critical review," *Journal of Dental Research*, 98, 8 (2019): 853–860.

14. Citizens for Public Justice, "Ending poverty in Canada." cpj.ca/election-2019-ending-poverty-canada/.

15. CAHS, "Improving access to oral health"; Carlos Quiñonez, *The Politics of Dental Care in Canada* (Toronto: Canadian Scholars Press, 2021): 176.

16. CAHS, "Improving access to oral health."

17. Michas, Frédéric, "Population to dentist ratio in Canada in 1997, 2005, and 2014, by province," *Statista*. statista.com/statistics/686403/population-to-dentist-ratio-in-canada-by-province/.

18. CAHS, "Improving access to oral health."

19. Margaret Whitley, "The high cost of food in Nunavut should shock all Canadians," *Huffington Post*, December 24, 2018. huffpost.com/entry/food-prices-canada-north_b_610841dbe4b052f1ce22188a; Leyland Cecco, "Dozens of Canada's First Nations lack drinking water: 'Unacceptable in a country so rich,'" *Guardian*, April 30,

2021; Grace Kyoon-Achan, Robert J. Schroth, Daniella DeMaré, Melina Sturym, Jeannette M. Edwards, Julianne Sanguins, Rhonda Campbell, Frances Chartrand, Mary Bertone and Michael EK Moffatt, "First Nations and Metis peoples' access and equity challenges with early childhood oral health: A qualitative study." *International Journal for Equity in Health,* 20, 1 (2021): 1–13.

20. Michèle Hébert, Chantal Czerednikow and Jonathan Lai, "People with developmental disabilities have a right to better dental care and less suffering," *Healthy Debate,* May 28, 2021. healthydebate. ca/2021/05/topic/developmental-disability-dentistry/.

21. Raul Garcia, Cynthia Cadoret and Michelle Henshaw, "Multicultural issues in oral health," *Dental Clinics of North America,* 52, 2 (2008): 319–332.

22. Catherine Carstairs and Ian Mosby, "Colonial extractions: Oral health care and Indigenous Peoples in Canada, 1945–79," *Canadian Historical Review,* 101, 2 (2020): 192–216.

23. Brandy Thompson, Peter Cooney, Herenia Lawrence, Vahid Ravaghi and Carlos Quiñonez, "The potential oral health impact of cost barriers to dental care: Findings from a Canadian population-based study," BMC *Oral Health,* 14, 1 (2014): 1–10; CAHS, "Improving access to oral health."

24. Carlos Quiñonez, "Why was dental care excluded from Canadian Medicare," *Network for Canadian Oral Health Research Working Papers Series,* 1, 1 (2013): 1–5; Hasan Sheikh, "CAEP dental care statement." *Canadian Journal of Emergency Medicine,* 22, 1 (2020): 36–39.

25. Alessandra Blaizot, Jean-Noël Vergnes, Samer Nuwwareh, Jacques Amar and Michel Sixou, "Periodontal diseases and cardiovascular events: Meta-analysis of observational studies," *International Dental Journal,* 59, 4 (2009): 197–209; George Taylor and Wenche Borgnakke, "Periodontal disease: Associations with diabetes, glycemic control and complications," *Oral Diseases,* 14, 3 (2008): 191–203; Daniel, Rajkumar, Subramanium Gokulanathan, Natarajan Shanmugasundaram, Mahalingam Lakshmigandhan and Thangavelu Kavin, "Diabetes and periodontal disease," *Journal of Pharmacy & Bioallied Sciences,* 4, 2 (2012): 280; Ahmad Haerian-Ardakani, Zia Eslami, Fahimeh Rashidi-Meibodi, Alireza Haerian,

Pantea Dallalnejad, Marjan Shekari, Amir Moein Taghavi and Solmaz Akbari, "Relationship between maternal periodontal disease and low birth weight babies," *Iranian Journal of Reproductive Medicine,* 11, 8 (2013): 625; S. Kellesarian, V. Malignaggi, C. Feng and F. Javed, "Association between obstructive sleep apnea and erectile dysfunction: A systematic review and meta-analysis," *International Journal of Impotence Research,* 30, 3 (2018): 129–140; Tzu-Hsien Lin, Chia-Chi Lung, Hsun-Pi Su, Jing-Yang Huang, Pei-Chieh Ko, Shiou-Rung Jan and Yi-Hua Sun, "Association between periodontal disease and osteoporosis by gender: A nationwide population-based cohort study," *Medicine,* 94, 7 (2015); Toyoko Morita, Yoko Ogawa, Koji Takada, Norihide Nishinoue, Yoshiyuki Sasaki, Masafumi Motohashi and Masao Maeno, "Association between periodontal disease and metabolic syndrome," *Journal of Public Health Dentistry,* 69, 4 (2009): 248–253; George Sfyroeras, Nikolaos Roussas, Vassileios G. Saleptsis, Christos Argyriou and Athanasios D. Giannoukas, "Association between periodontal disease and stroke," *Journal of Vascular Surgery,* 55, 4 (2012): 1178–1184.

26. Nadya, Marouf, Wenji Cai, Khalid N. Said, Hanin Daas, Hanan Diab, Venkateswara Rao Chinta, Ali Ait Hssain, Belinda Nicolau, Mariano Sanz and Faleh Tamimi, "Association between periodontitis and severity of COVID-19 infection: A case–control study," *Journal of Clinical Periodontology,* 48, 4 (2021): 483–491.

27. Yoneyama Takeyoshi, Mitsuyoshi Yoshida, Takashi Ohrui, Hideki Mukaiyama, Hiroshi Okamoto, Kanji Hoshiba, Shinichi Ihara, "Oral care reduces pneumonia in older patients in nursing homes," *Journal of the American Geriatrics Society,* 50, 3 (2002): 430–433; Jananni Muthu and Sivaramakrishnan Muthanandam, "Periodontitis and respiratory diseases: What does the recent evidence point to?," *Current Oral Health Reports,* 5 (2018): 63–69.

28. Terry Simpson, Ian Needleman, Sarah H. Wild, David R. Moles, and Edward J. Mills, "Treatment of periodontal disease for glycaemic control in people with diabetes," *Cochrane Database of Systematic Reviews,* 5 (2010).

29. Simpson, "Treatment of periodontal disease."

30. Francesco D'Aiuto, Derren Ready and Maurizio S. Tonetti,

"Periodontal disease and C-reactive protein-associated cardiovascular risk," *Journal of Periodontal Research*, 39, 4 (2004): 236–241.

31. Y. Matsuyama, H. Jürges, M. Dewey and S. Listl. "Causal effect of tooth loss on depression: Evidence from a population-wide natural experiment in the USA," *Epidemiology and Psychiatric Sciences*, 30 (2021).

32. C. Bedos, A. Levine and J. Brodeur, "How people on social assistance perceive, experience, and improve oral health," *Journal of Dental Research*, 88, 7 (2009): 653–657.

33. Bedos, "How people on social assistance"; Glen Hanson, Shawn McMillan, Kali Mower, Carter T. Bruett, Llely Duarte, Sri Koduri and Lilliam Pinzon, "Comprehensive oral care improves treatment outcomes in male and female patients with high-severity and chronic substance use disorders," *Journal of the American Dental Association*, 150, 7 (2019): 591–601.

34. Hanson, "Comprehensive oral care improves."

35. "Inequalities in oral health in Canada," Public Health Agency of Canada (2018). https://www.canada.ca/content/dam/phac-aspc/ documents/services/publications/science-research/phac-oral-health-en.pdf.

36. World Health Organization, "Oral health," (2022). who.int/ news-room/fact-sheets/detail/oral-health.

37. FDI World Dental Federation, "FDI's definition of oral health." https://www.fdiworlddental.org/fdis-definition-oral-health.

38. Government of Canada, *Canada Health Act*, Justice Laws Website R.S.C, C-6 (1985). laws-lois.justice.gc.ca/eng/acts/c-6/page-1. html.

39. Sonica Singhal, Carlos Quiñonez and Heather Manson, "Visits for nontraumatic dental conditions in Ontario's health care system," *Sage Journals*, 4, 1 (2018): 86–95.

40. "People pulling their own teeth highlights dental issues, says Mission," *CBC News*, March 20, 2018. cbc.ca/news/canada/ windsor/dental-changes-ontario-wynne-horwath-1.4583808.

41. Jacquie Maund, "Information on hospital emergency room visits for dental problems in Ontario," Ontario Oral Health Alliance, October 2014.

42. Sonical, "Visits for nontraumatic dental conditions."

43. Mario Brondani and Syed Ahmad, "The 1% of emergency room visits for non-traumatic dental conditions in British Columbia: Misconceptions about the numbers," *Canadian Journal of Public Health* (2017): 279.

44. "Barriers to dental care send thousands to emergency rooms for treatment," *Dentistry Today*, September 28, 2017. dentistrytoday. com/barriers-to-dental-care-send-thousands-to-emergency-rooms-for-treatment/.

45. Mitchell Levine, "Understanding how a dental infection may spread to the brain: Case report," *Journal of the Canadian Dental Association*, 79 (2013): 9.

46. Pei-Chun Chen, Ying-Chang Tung, Patricia W. Wu, Lung-Sheng Wu, Yu-Sheng Lin, Chee-Jen Chang, Suefang Kung and Pao-Hsien Chu, "Dental procedures and the risk of infective endocarditis," *Medicine,* 94, 43 (2015).

47. Karen Kleiss, "Girl, 9, nearly died from dental infection while on Alberta child welfare officials' watch: Report," *Edmonton Journal*, May 28, 2015. edmontonjournal.com/news/local-news/ girl-9-nearly-died-from-dental-infection-while-on-alberta-child-welfare-officials-watch-report.

48. Lauren Pelley, "Tooth issues can cause life-threatening conditions, advocates say, as feds move on dental care," CBC *News*, March 26, 2022. cbc.ca/news/health/dental-care-life-threatening-conditions-1.6397395?fbclid=IwAR1aHakyl26hZh0iX8cd34Fj gqn3_tTHF2rEIJBJDN3d_mdDuf5h4779iqc.

49. Gary Rine, "Sioux Lookout-area First Nations in 'dental crisis.' Health authority says," *TB News Watch*, June 16, 2021. tbnewswatch.com/local-news/sioux-lookout-area-first-nations-in-dental-crisis-health-authority-says-3880775.

50. Saskatchewan Health Authority, "Right care, right place, right time, right provider." https://www.rqhealth.ca/e-link-newsletter/ right-care-right-place-right-time-right-provider.

51. Sheikh, "CAEP Dental Care Statement."

52. "Global burden of bacterial antimicrobial resistance in 2019: A systematic analysis," *Lancet,* 399 (2022): 629–655.

53. Jim O'Neill, *Tackling Drug-Resistant Infections Globally: Final Report*

and Recommendations, Government of the United Kingdom (2016).

54. Sheikh, "CAEP Dental Care Statement."

55. Robert Schroth, Carlos Quiñonez, Luke Shwart, and Brandon Wagar, "Treating early childhood caries under general anesthesia: a national review of Canadian data," *Journal of the Canadian Dental Association,* 82, 20 (2016): 1–8.

56. Emma Tranter, "Wait-list for children's dental surgery in Nunavut has doubled to 1,000," *CBC News,* July 5, 2021. cbc.ca/news/canada/north/nunavut-dental-surgery-1.6090357.

57. Schroth, "Treating early childhood caries," table 1.

58. Michelle Ezer, N. Swoboda and D. Farkouh, "Early childhood caries: The dental disease of infants," *Journal Oral Health,* 100, 1 (2010).

59. George Acs, Gina Lodolini, Steven Kaminsky and George J. Cisneros, "Effect of nursing caries on body weight in a pediatric population," *Pediatric Dentistry,* 14, 5 (1992): 303.

60. Tranter, "Wait-list for children's dental."

61. King's College London, "Teeth hold the key to early diagnosis of eating disorders," (2018). kcl.ac.uk/news/teeth-hold-the-key-to-early-diagnosis-of-eating-disorders-4.

62. Paa-Kwesi Blankson, Francis Kwamin and Aaron Osei Asibey, "Screening at the dental office: An opportunity for bridging the gap in the early diagnosis of hypertension and diabetes in Ghana," *Annals of African Medicine,* 19, 1 (2020): 40–46; Centers for Disease Control and Prevention, "Oral Health Conditions," November 3, 2020. cdc.gov/oralhealth/conditions/index.html.

Chapter 2: The Structure of Dental Care

1. "Poll: Canadians are most proud of universal medicare," *CTV News,* November 25, 2012.

2. Carlos Quiñonez, "Why was dental care excluded from Canadian Medicare," *Network for Canadian Oral Health Research Working Papers Series,* 1, 1 (2013): 1–5.

3. Diarra Sourang and Aidan Worswick, "Cost estimate of a federal dental care program for uninsured Canadians," Office of the Parliamentary Budget Officer (2021): 2.

4. Sourang, "Cost estimate of a federal dental care," 2.

5. Malini Chari, "Comparing the magnitude of oral health inequality in Canada, United States and United Kingdom," (unpublished doctoral dissertation, University of Toronto, 2020): 21.

6. Richard Scheffler, *World Scientific Handbook of Global Health Economics and Public Policy (a 3-volume set)*, Vol. 3, (World Scientific, 2016): 83–121; Chantal Ramraj, Eleanor Weitzner, Rafael Figueiredo and Carlos Quiñonez, "A macroeconomic review of dentistry in Canada in the 2000s," *Journal of the Canadian Dental Association*, 80, 55 (2014).

7. Carlos Quiñonez, *The Politics of Dental Care in Canada* (Toronto: Canadian Scholars, 2021), table 1.1; D. Parkin and N. Devlin, "Measuring efficiency in dental care," *Advances in Health Economics* (2003): 143–66.

8. Carlos Quiñonez, "The political economy of dentistry in Canada," (doctoral dissertation, University of Toronto, 2009) 140.

9. Statistics Canada, "Health fact sheets: Dental care, 2018," September 16, 2019. 150.statcan.gc.ca/n1/pub/82-625-x/2019001/article/00010-eng.htm.

10. Laura Duncan and Ashley Bonner, "Effects of income and dental insurance coverage on need for dental care in Canada," *Journal of the Canadian Dental Association*, 80 (2014): 6.

11. Canadian Dental Association, "Findings: Ipsos Reid public opinion survey of dentists and the dental profession," August 10, 2010.

12. Armita Dehmoobadsharifabadi, Sonica Singhal and Carlos Quiñonez, "Investigating the "inverse care law" in dental care: A comparative analysis of Canadian jurisdictions," *Canadian Journal of Public Health*, 107, 6 (2016): 538-e544; Quiñonez, *Politics of Dental Care*, 13–14.

13. Statistics Canada, "Health fact sheets."

14. Quiñonez, *The Politics of Dental Care*, figure 2.16.

15. Don Taylor and Bradley Dow, "The rise of industrial unionism in Canada: A history of the CIO," Queen's University Industrial Relations Centre Archive Document 56 (1988): 28–31.

16. Quiñonez, "The politics of dental care," 20–21, figure 2.18.

17. Julia Kagan and Thomas Catalano, "Group Health Insurance," Investopedia, July 6, 2021. investopedia.com/terms/g/

group-health-insurance-plan.asp; Michael Law, Jillian Kratzer and Irfan Dhalla, "The increasing inefficiency of private health insurance in Canada," *Canadian Medical Association Journal*, 186: 12 (2014).

18. Sourang, "Cost estimate of a federal dental care," figure 1-2.

19. Meng Qingyue, Jia Liying and Yuan Beibei, "Cost-sharing mechanisms in health insurance schemes: A systematic review," The Alliance for Health Policy and Systems Research, WHO (2011): 1–76.

20. Safe. "What are the best dental insurance plans in Canada?" hellosafe.ca/en/health-insurance/dental-insurance; Jeremiah Hurley and Emmanuel Guindon, *Private Health Insurance in Canada*, Centre for Health Economics and Policy Analysis (2008).

21. Carlos Quiñonez and Paul Grootendorst, "Equity in dental care among Canadian households," *International Journal for Equity in Health*, 10, 1 (2011): 1–9.

22. Green Shield Canada, "GSC and community partners launch new reports uncovering the social impact of oral health," April 7, 2022. greenshield.ca/en-ca/blog/post/gsc-and-community-partners-launch-new-reports-uncovering-the-social-impact-of-oral-health.

23. Ake Blomqvist and Frances Woolley, "Filling the cavities: Improving the efficiency and equity of Canada's dental care system," CD Howe Institute Commentary 510 (2018).

24. Britannica. "Dentistry: Types of Practice." britannica.com/science/dentistry/Ancillary-dental-fields.

25. David Rosenthal, "Non-dental ownership of dental practice," The Professional Advisory for Dental Professionals, February 23, 2013. professionaladvisory.ca/content/non-dental-ownership-of-dental-practice.

26. Dental Hygiene Canada, "Independent Dental Hygienists." https://www.dentalhygienecanada.ca/dhcanada/DHCanada/Your_Dental_Hygienist/Independent_Dental_Hygienists.aspx.

27. Denturist Association of Canada. "About denturism: Denturism in Canada." https://www.denturist.org/about.html.

28. Fran Richardson, "The Canadian view of self-regulation," RHD *Magazine* (2004); Denturist Association of Canada, "About denturism."

29. Dental Career Options, "Practice Models." https://

dentalcareeroptions.ca/practice-models/.

30.   CDA (Canadian Dental Association), "Economic realities of practice." Cda-adc.ca/en/services/internationallytrained/economic/.

31.   Royal College of Dental Surgeons of Ontario, "Fees & charges." rcdso.org/en-ca/patients-general-public/resources-for-patients/fees.

32.   Gavin Prout, "Why your dental fee guide is important and how to understand it," Special Benefits Insurance Services. sbis.ca/why-your-dental-fee-guide-is-important-and-how-to-understand-it.html.

33   Gavin Prout, "Who regulates dental care and billing in Canada?" Special Benefits Insurance Services. sbis.ca/regulates-dental-care-billing-canada.html.

34.   Leigh Doyle, "A look at the drivers for curbing rising dental costs," *Benefits Canada*, October 12, 2018. benefitscanada.com/news/bencan/a-look-at-the-drivers-for-curbing-rising-dental-costs/.

35.   "Albertans pay more for dental care, government review finds," *Calgary Herald*, December 8, 2016.

36.   "New guide recommends dental fees in Alberta drop 8.5%," CBC *News*, November 22, 2017.

37.   Quiñonez, "The Politics of Dental Care in Canada," 162, figure 3.9.

38.   Green Shield Canada, "GSC and community partners."

39.   Stefan Listl and Martin Chalkley, "Provider payment bares teeth: Dentist reimbursement and the use of check-up examinations," *Social Science & Medicine*, 111 (2014): 110–116.

40.   Ferris Jabr, "The truth about dentistry," *The Atlantic*, May 2019. theatlantic.com/magazine/archive/2019/05/the-trouble-with-dentistry/586039/.

41.   Blomqvist, "Filling the cavities," 14.

42.   Canadian Dental Association, "Findings."

43.   Abdulrahman Ghoneim, "How does competition affect the clinical decision-making of dentists in Ontario?" (doctoral dissertation, University of Toronto, 2018); Quiñonez, "The politics of dental care in Canada," 228.

44.   Blomqvist, "Filling the cavities," 16; Quiñonez, "The politics of dental care in Canada," 229.

45.   Listl, "Provider payment bares teeth."

46. Wen-Chen Tsai, Pei-Tseng Kung and Wei-Chieh Chang, "Influences of market competition on dental care utilization under the global budget payment system," *Community Dentistry and Oral Epidemiology,* 35, 6 (2007): 459–464.

47. Jostein Grytten, "Payment systems and incentives in dentistry," *Community Dentistry and Oral Epidemiology,* 45, 1 (2017): 1–11.

48. Abdulrahman Ghoneim, Bonnie Yu, Herenia Lawrence, Michael Glogauer, Ketan Shankardass and Carlos Quiñonez, "What influences the clinical decision-making of dentists? A cross-sectional study," *PLoS One,* 15, 6 (2020).

49. Brigitte Bigras, Johnson Bradford, Ellen. BeGole and Christopher Wenckus, "Differences in clinical decision making: A comparison between specialists and general dentists," *Oral Surgery, Oral Medicine, Oral Pathology, Oral Radiology, and Endodontology,* 106, 1 (2008): 139–144.

50. "Dentists vary widely on diagnosis and cost, CBC Marketplace finds," *CBC News,* October 18, 2012. cbc.ca/news/canada/dentists-vary-widely-on-diagnosis-and-cost-cbc-marketplace-finds-1.1279371.

51. "Dentists vary widely on diagnosis," *CBC News.*

52. Joseph Stromberg, "How to avoid getting ripped off by the dentist," *Vox,* August 12, 2014. vox.com/2014/8/12/5951321/dentistry-fraud-treatments-products; E. Ertas, A Aksoy, A. Turla, E. Karaarslan, B. Karaarsla, A. Aydin and A. Eken, "Human brain mercury levels related to exposure to amalgam fillings," *Human & Experimental Toxicology,* 33, 8 (2–13): 873–877.

53. Quiñonez, "The politics of dental care," 208–209; Mary Otto, *Teeth: The Story of Beauty, Inequality, and the Struggle for Oral Health in America* (New York: The New Press, 2017): 22.

54. Canadian Dental Association, "Findings."

55. Evan Frisbee, "Dental Veneers," WebMD, July 20, 2020. webmd.com/oral-health/guide/veneers.

56. "Dentists vary widely on diagnosis," *CBC News.*

57. Gordon J. Christensen, "I have had enough! By Gordon J. Christensen, DDS, MSD, PhD," *Dental Town* (2003). https://www.dentaltown.com/magazine/article/455/i-have-had-enough.

58. Tracey Adams, *Regulating Professions* (Toronto: University of

Toronto Press, 2018): 6.

59.   Adams, *Regulating Professions*, 85.

60.   Andrea MacGregor. "Conflicts of interest in self-regulating health professions regulators, 2021," *Dalhousie Law Journal* (2021).

61.   Adams, *Regulating Professions*, 4; see also Richard Abel, *English Lawyers between Market and State: The Politics of Professionalism* (London: Oxford University Press, 2003).

62.   Adams, *Regulating Professions*, 22–23.

63.   "Dental fraud," CBC *Marketplace* (1998). https://www.cbc.ca/player/play/2293999023.

64.   *An Inquiry into the Performance of the College of Dental Surgeons of British Columbia and the Health Professions Act*, Professional Standards Authority (2018); Bethany Lindsay, "Rip up current system and start over, recommends review of B.C.'s professional health colleges," CBC *News* (2019). https://www.cbc.ca/news/canada/british-columbia/bc-health-professional-regulation-report-1.5094180.

Chapter 3: The History of Dental Care in Canada

1.   Tracey Adams, *A Dentist and a Gentleman: Gender and the Rise of Dentistry in Canada* (Toronto: University of Toronto Press, 2000), 19–20.

2.   Donald Gullett, *A History of Dentistry in Canada* (Toronto: University of Toronto Press, 1971), 93.

3.   Gullett, *A History of Dentistry in Canada*, 12, 19.

4.   Gullett, *A History of Dentistry in Canada*, 22–25.

5.   Adams, *A Dentist and a Gentleman*, 27–34.

6.   Adams, *A Dentist and a Gentleman*, 36.

7.   Adams, *A Dentist and a Gentleman*, 77–79.

8.   Tracey Adams, *Regulating Professions* (Toronto: University of Toronto Press, 2018), 242.

9.   Adams, *Regulating Professions,* 114.

10.   Adams, *Regulating Professions,* 134

11.   Robert Gidney and Winnifred Millar, *Professional Gentlemen: The Professions in Nineteenth-Century Ontario* (Toronto: University of Toronto Press, 1994), 217.

12. Adams, *A Dentist and a Gentleman*, 40.
13. Adams, *A Dentist and a Gentleman*, 72.
14. Gullett, *A History of Dentistry in Canada*, 74.
15. Gullett, *A History of Dentistry in Canada*, 127.
16. James Struthers, "The Great Depression in Canada," *Canadian Encyclopedia*, July 11, 2013. thecanadianencyclopedia.ca/en/article/great-depression.
17. "Post World War II economic boom," University of Waterloo: Special Collections and Archives. uwaterloo.ca/library/special-collections-archives/exhibits/doerr-dare-story-canadian-business/post-world-war-ii-economic-boom; CBC Learning, "The fight for Medicare." cbc.ca/history/EPISCONTENTSE1EP15CH2PA4LE.html.
18. Carlos Quiñonez, "Why was dental care excluded from Canadian Medicare," *Network for Canadian Oral Health Research*, 1, 1 (2013): 2.
19. Lorne Brown and Doug Taylor, "The birth of Medicare: From Saskatchewan's breakthrough to Canada wide coverage," *Canadian Dimension*, July 3, 2012. canadiandimension.com/articles/view/the-birth-of-medicare.
20. Bruce Campbell and Greg Marchildon, *Completing Tommy's vision: Medicare's future*, Canadian Centre for Policy Alternatives, November 19, 2007. policyalternatives.ca/publications/commentary/completing-tommys-vision
21. Campbell, *Completing Tommy's vision.*
22. Brown, "The birth of Medicare."
23. Colleen Fuller and Susan Rosenthal, *Caring for Profit: How Corporations Are Taking Over Canada's Health Care System* (Vancouver: New Star Books, 1999): 48–50.
24. Brian Bergman, "Emmett Hall (obituary)." *Canadian Encyclopedia*, Mar 17 2003. thecanadianencyclopedia.ca/en/article/emmett-hall-obituary.
25. Leake, James L. "Why do we need an oral health care policy in Canada?" *Journal of the Canadian Dental Association*, 72, 4 (2006): 317.
26. Fuller, *Caring for Profit*, 59.
27. Fuller, *Caring for Profit*, 25.

28. Brown, "The birth of Medicare."

29. Brown, "The birth of Medicare."

30. Stan Rands, *Privilege and Policy: A History of Community Clinics in Saskatchewan* (Edmonton: Canadian Plains Research Centre Press, 2012): 76.

31. Leo Panitch, *The Canadian State: Political Economy and Political Power* (University of Toronto Press, 1977): 320.

32. Brown, "The birth of Medicare."

33. John Morley, "Co-operative Commonwealth Federation (CCF)," *Canadian Enyclopedia*, March 26, 2021. thecanadianencyclopedia. ca/en/article/co-operative-commonwealth-federation.

34. Brown, "The birth of Medicare."

35. Brown, "The birth of Medicare."

36. Janice Tyrwhitt and Douglas Marshall, "Why Canadian kids get a rotten deal in dental care," *Macleans*, January 1, 1967.

37. Author unknown ,"Self-interested education in prevention," *Journal of the Canadian Dental Association*, 42 (1976): 56.

38. National Committee for Mental Hygiene (Canada), "Study of the distribution of medical care and public health services in Canada," (1939). archive.org/details/studyofdistribut0000unse.

39. Tyrwhitt, "Why Canadian kids get a rotten deal."

40. Gullett, *A History of Dentistry in Canada*, 160–164.

41. Gullett, *A History of Dentistry in Canada*, 223.

42. E.J. Ryan EJ, "National health program," *Journal of the Canadian Dental Association*, 5 (1939): 562, cited in Carlos Quiñonez, *The Politics of Dental Care in Canada* (Toronto, Canadian Scholars Press, 2021): 36.

43. Carlos Quiñonez, *The Political Economy of Dentistry in Canada* (University of Toronto Press, 2009): 122.

44. Andrew Longhurst, "How (and how much) doctors are paid: Why it matters," *Policy Note*, January 15, 2019. policynote.ca/how-and-how-much-doctors-are-paid-why-it-matters/.

45. Donald Gullet, "Some phases of dental health insurance in Canada," *Journal of the Canadian Dental Association*, 10 (1944): 9.

46. Brandy Thompson, Peter Cooney, Herenia Lawrence, Vahid Ravaghi and Carlos Quiñonez, "The potential oral health impact of cost barriers to dental care: Findings from a Canadian

population-based study." BMC *Oral Health,* 14, 1 (2014): 1–10.

47. Joan O'Connell, Diane Brunson, Theresa Anselmo and Patrick W. Sullivan, "Costs and savings associated with community water fluoridation programs in Colorado," *Preventing Chronic Disease,* 2 (2005): 6.

48. Richard Lyons, "End of most tooth decay predicted for near future," *New York Times,* 1983.

49. Quiñonez, *The Political Economy of Dentistry in Canada,* 207–208.

50. C. Castaldi, "Children's dental health plan," *Journal of the Canadian Dental Association,* 34 (1968): 235–236.

51. CBC Learning, "The fight for Medicare."

52. Government of Canada. Department of National Health and Welfare, *Ad Hoc Committee on Dental Auxiliaries: Report* (1970).

53. Garry Ewart, "The Saskatchewan Children's Dental Plan: Is it time for renewal?" (dissertation, University of Regina, 2010): 25–26. https://saskohc.ca/images/pdf/hdphis/hdphis2.pdf.

54. Ewart, "The Saskatchewan Children's Dental Plan," 40.

55. Ewart, "The Saskatchewan Children's Dental Plan," 27.

56. Ewart, "The Saskatchewan Children's Dental Plan," 27.

57. Ewart, "The Saskatchewan Children's Dental Plan," 27–28.

58. Ewart, "The Saskatchewan Children's Dental Plan," 28–29.

59. Ewart, "The Saskatchewan Children's Dental Plan," 56–57.

60. Ewart, "The Saskatchewan Children's Dental Plan," 33.

61. Saskatchewan Dental Therapists Association, *History of dental therapy in Saskatchewan.* sdta.ca/history.html; Saskatchewan Dental Therapists Association, "Legislation." sdta.ca/legislation.html.

62. Kavita Mathu-Muju, Jay W. Friedman and David A. Nash. "Saskatchewan's school-based dental program staffed by dental therapists: A retrospective case study," *Journal of Public Health Dentistry,* 77, 1 (2017): 78–85.

63. Mathu-Muju, "Saskatchewan's school-based dental program," 80.

64. Ewart, "The Saskatchewan Children's Dental Plan," 55; "Saskatchewan Dental Therapists Association, "History of dental therapy in Saskatchewan."

65. Saskatchewan: Department of Public Health, *Saskatchewan Dental Plan: A Quality Evaluation of Specific Dental Services Provided by the Saskatchewan Dental Plan — Final Report* (1976).

66. Mathu-Muju, "Saskatchewan's school-based dental program," figure 3; Quiñonez, *The Political Economy of Dentistry in Canada,* 103.

67. Stephanie Rezansoff, "SHDP: An experiment in success that failed," *Saskatchewan Economic Journal* (1997): 1–9.

68. Rezansoff, " SHDP: An experiment in success that failed," table 2.

69. Rezansoff, " SHDP: An experiment in success that failed," table 4.

70. Rezansoff, " SHDP: An experiment in success that failed," 1–9.

71. Ewart, "The Saskatchewan Children's Dental Plan," 49.

72. Ewart, "The Saskatchewan Children's Dental Plan," 123.

73. Ewart, "The Saskatchewan Children's Dental Plan," 58, 62–63.

74. Douglas Campbell, "Dental programs," *Moose Jaw Times-Herald,* August 20, 1976.

75. Allan Blakeney, Provincial Archives of Saskatchewan, 565, 3. 347.

76. Ewart, "The Saskatchewan Children's Dental Plan," 64.

77. Ewart, "The Saskatchewan Children's Dental Plan," 77–78.

78. Ewart, "The Saskatchewan Children's Dental Plan," 79; Dennis Gruending, *Promises to Keep: A Political Biography of Allan Blakeney* (Saskatoon: Western Producer Prairie Books, 1990).

79. Dale Eisler, "Dental plan cost report denied," *Regina Leader Post,* June 20, 1987: 4.

80. Rezansoff, " SHDP: An experiment in success that failed," 5–8.

81. Ewart, "The Saskatchewan Children's Dental Plan," 151.

82. Ewart, "The Saskatchewan Children's Dental Plan," 155.

83. Ewart, "The Saskatchewan Children's Dental Plan," 86–87.

84. Saskatchewan Legislative Assembly, *Hansard Debates,* 1, 2 (1987): 14–15, 19, 27 & 30–32.

85. "Gov't dental gear gathers dust," *Regina Leader Post,* May 27, 1989: 4; "Leftover dental equipment said headed for scrap heap," *Regina Leader Post,* June 13, 1989: 4.

86. Randy Burton, "Blakeney says PCs are killing the dream," *Saskatoon Phoenix,* June 22, 1987: 3.

87. Mark Merryfield, "A survey of periodontal conditions in adolescents enrolled in the Saskatchewan Health Dental Plan," Saskatchewan Health Dental Plan, (1983).

88. Victoria Leck and Glen Randall, "The rise and fall of dental therapy in Canada: A policy analysis and assessment of equity of access

to oral health care for Inuit and First Nations communities," *International Journal for Equity in Health,* 16, 1 (2017): 1–10.

89.   Mike Rudyk, "Yukon scales back in-school dental program," *CBC News,* December 12, 2019. cbc.ca/news/canada/north/ yukon-school-dental-program-1.5393424.

90.   "USask collaboration establishes first dental therapy degree program in Canada," *University of Saskatchewan* (2022). https:// news.usask.ca/articles/colleges/2022/usask-collaboration-establishes-first-dental-therapy-degree-program-in-canada.php.

Chapter 4: Public Dental Programs

1.   Colleen Fuller and Susan Rosenthal, *Caring for Profit: How Corporations Are Taking Over Canada's Health Care System* (Vancouver: New Star Books, 1999) 59; James L. Leake, "Why do we need an oral health care policy in Canada?" *Journal of the Canadian Dental Association,* 72: 4 (2006) 317; Elisabeth McClymont, "Dental care in Canada: the need for incorporation into publicly funded health care," *University of British Columbia Medical Journal,* 7, 1.

2.   Carlos Quiñonez, "Why was dental care excluded from Canadian Medicare?" *Network for Canadian Oral Health Research,* 1, 1 (2013): 2.

3.   Jason Chung, "Canadians can be smug about our health care system when public coverage extends to dental care," *CBC News,* June 15, 2017. cbc.ca/news/opinion/public-dental-care-1.4160243.

4.   Carlos Quiñonez, "The political economy of dentistry in Canada" (doctoral dissertation, University of Toronto): 164.

5.   Jodi Shaw and Julie Farmer, *An Environmental Scan of Publicly Financed Dental Care in Canada: 2015 Update* (2015). https:// caphd.ca/wp-content/uploads/2022/06/FINAL-2015-Environmental-Scan-ENGLISH-16-Feb-16.pdf.

6.   Quiñonez, "The political economy of dentistry," 84.

7.   Shaw, *An Environmental Scan,* figure 5.

8.   Ian Mosby and Catherine Carstairs, "Federal policies undermine Indigenous dental health," *Policy Options,* October 5, 2018. policyoptions.irpp.org/magazines/october-2018/

federal-policies-undermine-indigenous-dental-health/.

9.   Tom Lange, "Polishing-up for the election: Lessons from Indigenous dental care," YYC Policy, October 10, 2019. yycpolicy. org/blog/2019/10/10/polishing-up-for-the-election-lessons-from-indigenous-dental-care; Canadian Institute for Health Information, "National health expenditure trends," November 4, 2021. www.cihi. ca/en/national-health-expenditure-trends.

10. Shaw, *An Environmental Scan,* figures 37, 38.

11. Laura Osman, "Budget 2022 makes good on dental care, but little in new health spending," CTV News, April 7, 2022. ctvnews.ca/ politics/budget-2022-makes-good-on-dental-care-but-little-in-new-health-spending-1.5852870.

12. Carlos Quiñonez, *The Politics of Dental Care in Canada* (Toronto: Canadian Scholars Press, 2021) table 3.1; Shaw, *An Environmental Scan.*

13. Åke Blomqvist and Farnces Woolley, "Improving the efficiency and equity of Canada's dental care system," CD Howe Institute 510 (May 2018); Christopher Lange, "Comprehensive dental care in Canada: The choice between denticaid and denticare," *School of Public Policy Publications,* 13, 22 (September 2020): figure 1.

14. Josh Sherman, "These Ontario experts are calling for universal dental care," TVO, May 11, 2021. tvo.org/article/these-ontario-experts-are-calling-for-universal-dental-care; Luke Hendry, "Health board to call for comprehensive low-income dental care," *The Intelligencer,* February 2, 2022. intelligencer.ca/news/ health-board-to-call-for-comprehensive-low-income-dental-care; Nicole Kleinsteuber, "Board of health calls on province for oral care funding," *Inquinte,* February 1, 2022. inquinte.ca/story/ board-of-health-calls-on-province-for-oral-care-funding/direct.

15. Carlos Quiñonez, Rafael Figueiredo and David Locker, "Canadian dentists' opinions on publicly financed dental care," *Journal of Public Health Dentistry,* 69, 2 (2009): 64–73.

16. Quiñonez, "Canadian dentists' opinions on publicly financed"; Shaw, *An Environmental Scan,* 11–12.

17. René Bruemmer, "Quebec dentists to withdraw en masse from public health-care system Friday," *Montreal Gazette,* February 14, 2020. montrealgazette.com/news/local-news/

quebec-dentists-to-withdraw-en-masse-from-public-health-care-system-Friday.

18. Lange, "Comprehensive dental care in Canada," figure 1.

19. Ontario: Ministry of Health, "Teeth cleaning, check-ups and dental treatment for kids," September 4, 2014. ontario.ca/page/get-dental-care.

20. Shaw, *An Environmental Scan.*

21. Blomqvist, "Improving the efficiency and equity."

22. Krystle Maki, "Neoliberal deviants and surveillance: Welfare recipients under the watchful eye of Ontario Works," *Surveillance & Society,* 9 (2011).

23. British Columbia, "Dental coverage." 2.gov.bc.ca/gov/content/family-social-supports/income-assistance/on-assistance/supplements/dental.

24. Newfoundland Labrador Canada: Health and Community Services, "Dental services: General info." gov.nl.ca/hcs/dentalservices/general-info/.

25. Joan Rush, "Help! Teeth hurt: Government's obligation to provide timely access to dental treatment to B.C. adults who have developmental disabilities: A legal analysis," self-published.

26. Keith Da Silva, Julie Farmer and Carlos Quiñonez, "Access to oral health care for individuals with developmental disabilities: An umbrella review," Federal-Provincial-Territorial Dental Directors Working Group (2017).

27. Toronto, "Healthy smiles ontario program." toronto.ca/311/knowledgebase/kb/docs/articles/public-health/dental-and-oral-health-services/healthy-smiles-ontario-program.html#:~:text=On October 1%2C 2010 the,eligible children 17 and under.

28. Canadian Dental Hygienists Association, "National oral health care for seniors." cdha.ca/cdha/The_Profession_folder/Policy__Advocacy_folder/Oral_Health_Care_for_Seniors/CDHA/The_Profession/Policy_Advocacy/Oral_Health_Care_for_Seniors.aspx.

29. Lange, "Comprehensive dental care in Canada," figure 1.

30. Ontario: Minister of Health, "Dental care for low-income seniors," November 20, 2019. ontario.ca/page/dental-care-low-income-seniors.

31. "A 2-month wait to fix his 2 front teeth: The problem with the Ontario seniors dental program," CBC *News*, January 20, 2020. cbc.ca/news/canada/windsor/seniors-dental-program-ontario-windsor-teeth-1.5433138.

32. Hendry, "Health board to call for comprehensive"; Kleinsteuber, "Board of health calls"; Isaac Callan, "Underfunded system in Peel failing seniors, again," *The Pointer*, November 11, 2021. thepointer.com/article/2021-11-11/underfunded-system-in-peel-failing-seniors-again.

33. Statistics Canada, "Financial information of universities and degree-granting colleges, 2015/2016." 150.statcan.gc.ca/n1/daily-quotidien/170713/dq170713c-eng.htm; ADEA, "Canadian dental schools." cqrcengage.com/adea/canadentalschools; Schulich Medicine and Dentistry "Treatment Costs." schulich.uwo.ca/dentistry/dental_clinics/becoming_a_patient/treatment_costs.html.

34. Canadian Dental Association, "Dental care FAQs." cda-adc.ca/en/oral_health/faqs/dental_care_faqs.asp.

35. Quiñonez, "Canadian dentists' opinions on publicly financed."

36. Faculty of Dentistry, "In the community." dal.ca/faculty/dentistry/about/community.html; University of Alberta, "New partnership aims to improve access to care." ualberta.ca/school-of-dentistry/about-us/dentistrynews/2020/november/mna-partner.html; David Leblanc, "Transformational partnership increases access to community dental care," McGill Dentistry, November 4, 2021. mcgill.ca/dentistry/article/faculty-news/transformational-partnership-increases-access-community-dental-care; Harinder Sandhu and David Mock, "Dental schools are committed to increasing access to care." *Journal of the Canadian Dental Association,* 76 (2010): 5.

37. Quiñonez, *The Politics of Dental Care in Canada*, 92–93.

38. Quiñonez, *The Politics of Dental Care in Canada*, table 2.5.

39. Government of Canada, "Dental Officer." forces.ca/en/career/dental-officer/.

40. Correctional Service Canada, "Beyond the fence: A virtual tour of a Canadian penitentiary —health care centre," February 1, 2015. csc-scc.gc.ca/csc-virtual-tour/15-eng.shtml.

41. "CDA presents to senate committee on dental care in correctional facilities," CDA *Essentials*, 3 (2019) 15.

42. Glen Hanson, Shawn McMillan, Kali Mower, Carter T. Bruett, Llely Duarte, Sri Koduri and Lilliam Pinzon, "Comprehensive oral care improves treatment outcomes in male and female patients with high-severity and chronic substance use disorders," *Journal of the American Dental Association*, 150, 7 (2019): 591–601.

43. Leeann Donnelly, Ruth Martin and Mario Brondani, "Perceived oral health and access to care among men with a history of incarceration," *Canadian Dental Hygiene Journal*, 53, 3 (2019) 157–165.

44. Government of Canada, "Interim federal health program: About the program," September 13, 2017. canada.ca/en/immigration-refugees-citizenship/services/refugees/help-within-canada/health-care/interim-federal-health-program.html.

45. Government of Canada, "Interim federal health program: Who is eligible," December 21, 2020. canada.ca/en/immigration-refugees-citizenship/services/refugees/help-within-canada/health-care/interim-federal-health-program/eligibility.html.

46. Government of Canada, "Interim federal health program: What is covered," September 10, 2021. canada.ca/en/immigration-refugees-citizenship/services/refugees/help-within-canada/health-care/interim-federal-health-program/coverage-summary.html.

47. Nazik Nurelhuda, Mark Keboa, Herenia Lawrence, Belinda Nicolau and Mary Macdonald, "Advancing our understanding of dental care pathways of refugees and asylum seekers in Canada: A qualitative study," *International Journal of Environmental and Research and Public Health*, 18: 16 (2021).

48. "Non-Insured Health Benefits and Aboriginals," November 2010. https://www.aboriginalsexualhealth.ca/documents/NonInsuredHealthBenefits.pdf.

49. Government of Canada, "Benefits and services under the Non-Insured Health Benefits program," December 20, 2019. sac-isc.gc.ca/eng/1572545056418/1572545109296.

50. Government of Canada, "Dental benefits guide: Non-Insured Health Benefits program," September 23, 2021. sac-isc.gc.ca/eng/1579538771806/1579538804799#a8642.

51. Mosby, "Federal policies undermine Indigenous dental health."
52. Government of Canada, "Dental benefits guide for First Nations and Inuit" September 23, 2021. sac-isc.gc.ca/eng/1579538771806/1579538804799.
53. Mosby, "Federal policies undermine Indigenous dental health."
54. John Paul Tasker, "Ottawa spent $110k in legal fees fighting First Nations girl over $6k dental procedure," CBC News, September 29, 2017. cbc.ca/news/politics/health-canada-legal-fees-first-nations-girl-dental-coverage-1.4310224.
55. Lange, "Polishing-up for the Election."
56. Shari Narine, "AFN tackling the dwindling benefits of NIHB," Wind Speaker, February 2014, 18. data2.archives.ca/e/e449/e011200926.pdf.
57. Tripartite First Nations Health Plan, "Healthy smiles for life: BC's First Nations and Aboriginal oral health strategy" (2014). https://www.fnha.ca/about/news-and-events/news/healthy-smiles-for-life-bcs-first-nations-and-aboriginal-oral-health-strategy.
58. Meaghan Ketcheson, "New Manitoba senator says federal dental program for First Nations, Inuit communities isn't working," CBC News, February 7, 2018. cbc.ca/news/canada/manitoba/senator-mary-jane-mccallum-first-nations-dental-care-1.4524506.
59. Catharine Tunney, "Liberals agree to launch dental care program in exchange for NDP support," CBC News, March 22, 2022. cbc.ca/news/politics/trudeu-jagmeet-singh-deal-government-1.6393021.
60. PBO (Office of the Parliamentary Budget Officer), "Cost estimate of a federal dental care program for uninsured Canadians" (October 2020).
61. Tunney, "Liberals agree to launch dental care program."
62. PBO, "Cost estimate of a federal dental."
63. Mark Creighton, "Cost of a dental care plan for Canadians," Office of the Parliamentary Budget Officer, June 16, 2022.
64. Osman, "Budget 2022 makes good on dental care."
65. Natasha Bulowski, "Liberals, NDP unveil 'single biggest expansion of public health care in 60 years," Canada's National Observer (2022).
66. Government of Canada: Department of Finance Canada, "Making dental care more affordable: The Canada dental benefit." canada.ca/en/department-finance/news/2022/09/

making-dental-care-more-affordable-the-canada-dental-benefit.
html.

67. Government of Canada, *Canada Health Act*, Justice Laws Website
     R.S.C, C-6 (1985). laws-lois.justice.gc.ca/eng/acts/c-6/page-1.
     html.

68. Quiñonez, *The Politics of Dental Care in Canada*, 102–103.

69. Alberta Government, "Alberta Health Care Insurance Plan:
     Schedule of oral and maxillofacial surgery benefits [2019]." open.
     alberta.ca/publications/schedule-of-dental-benefits.

70. Reginald Goodday, Susan Bourque and Pember Edwards,
     "Objective and subjective outcomes following maxillomandibular
     advancement surgery for treatment of patients with extremely
     severe obstructive sleep apnea (apnea-hypopnea index> 100),"
     Journal of Oral and Maxillofacial Surgery, 74, 3 (2016): 583–589.

71. Blomqvist, "Improving the efficiency and equity"; Lange,
     "Comprehensive dental care in Canada"; CCPA (Canadian Centre
     for Policy Alternatives), "Putting our money where our mouth
     is: The future of dental care in Canada" (April 2011); Canadian
     Association of Public Health Dentistry, "Roadmap to universal
     dental care" (September 2020); Arlene King, *Oral Health – More
     Than Just Cavities: A Report by Ontario's Chief Medical Officer of
     Health* (April 27, 2012) 20. https://www.health.gov.on.ca/en/
     common/ministry/publications/reports/oral_health/oral_health.
     aspx.

72. Lange, "Comprehensive dental care in Canada."

73. CCPA, "Putting our money where our mouth is."

74. "Canadian dental coverage should focus on existing programs, says
     dentist group," *CityNews*, March 23, 2022. ottawa.citynews.ca/
     local-news/canadian-dental-coverage-should-focus-on-existing-
     programs-says-dentist-group-5188421.

75. CCPA, "Putting our money where our mouth is."

76. Carlos Quiñonez, "Dentistry in Alberta: Time for a checkup?"
     The Parkland Institute (2020) 32; Canadian Association of Public
     Health Dentistry, "Roadmap to universal dental care in Canada:
     Submission to the House of Commons standing committee on
     health" (2020): 4–5.

77. Lange, "Comprehensive dental care in Canada," 1.

78. Thomas Lange, "Starting from scratch: A micro-costing analysis for public dental care in Canada," *The School of Public Policy Publications,* 13 (2020).

79. Lange, "Starting from scratch"; Total Orthodontics, "What is the IOTN." https://www.dentalnotebook.com/iotn/.

80. Lange, "Starting from scratch."

81. Lange, "Comprehensive dental care in Canada," 6.

82. PBO, "Cost estimate of a federal dental."

83. PBO, "Cost estimate of a federal dental."

84. Osman, "Budget 2022 makes good on dental care."

85. Government of Canada, "Chapter 6: Strong public health care," April 7, 2022. budget.gc.ca/2022/report-rapport/chap6-en.html.

86. PBO, "Cost estimate of a federal dental," 2, 7.

87. Lange, "Comprehensive dental care in Canada," 1.

88. Lange, "Comprehensive dental care in Canada."

89. PBO, "Cost estimate of a federal dental," 7; Lange, "Comprehensive dental care in Canada," 2.

90. Lange, "Starting from scratch."

91. Lange, "Starting from scratch."

92. CCPA, "Putting our money where our mouth is," 15.

93. Quiñonez, "Dentistry in Alberta," 34.

94. CCPA, "Putting our money where our mouth is," 12.

95. "NDP pushing for dental care plan for households earning less than $90k," *VOCM* (May 9, 2021); Sherman, "These Ontario experts are calling for universal dental care."

96. Kevin Payne and Brandon Doucet, "Luxury bones — why we need universal dental care, and why it needs to be public," *Nova Scotia Advocate*, September 19, 2021. nsadvocate.org/2021/09/19/luxury-bones-why-we-need-universal-dental-care-and-why-it-needs-to-be-public/.

97. Jacques Gallant, "Liberal-NDP dental plan would benefit millions of Canadians," *Toronto Star*, March 22, 2022. thestar.com/politics/federal/2022/03/22/liberal-ndp-dental-plan-would-benefit-millions-of-canadians.html.

98. Lange, "Comprehensive dental care in Canada," 1.

99. Lange, "Comprehensive dental care in Canada," 20.

100. Eric Schneider, Arnav Shah, Michelle Doty, Roosa Tikkanen,

Katherine Fields and Reginald Williams II, *Mirror, Mirror 2021: Reflecting Poorly,* The Commonwealth Fund, August 4, 2021. commonwealthfund.org/publications/fund-reports/2021/aug/mirror-mirror-2021-reflecting-poorly.

101. D. Parkin and N. Devlin, "Measuring efficiency in dental care," *Advances in Health Economics* (2003): 143–166; Let's 8020, "8020 Promotion Foundation — Outline of its objectives and operations." https://www.8020zaidan.or.jp/english/; Takashi Zaitsu, Tomoya Saito and Yoko Kawaguchi, "The oral healthcare system in Japan," *Healthcare,* 6, 3, (2018): table 3.

102. Fumiaki Shinsho, "New strategy for better geriatric oral health in Japan: 80/20 movement and Healthy Japan 21," *International Dental Journal* 51 (2001): 200–206; Sachiko Ono, Miho Ishimaru, Hayato Yamana, Kojiro Morita, Yosuke Ono, Hiroki Matsui and Hideo Yasunaga, "Enhanced oral care and health outcomes among nursing facility residents: Analysis using the national long-term care database in Japan," *Journal of Post Acute and Long Term Care Medicine,* 1, 18 (2017): 277.

103. Joseph Lim, "8020 Campaign," *Panay News,* June 12, 2021. panaynews.net/8020-campaign/.

104. Blomqvist, "Improving the efficiency and equity."

105. Quiñonez, "Why was dental care excluded," 3.

106. Yoneyama Takeyoshi, Mitsuyoshi Yoshida, Takashi Ohrui, Hideki Mukaiyama, Hiroshi Okamoto, Kanji Hoshiba, Shinichi Ihara, "Oral care reduces pneumonia in older patients in nursing homes," *Journal of the American Geriatrics Society,* 50, 3 (2002).

107. Raj Desai, "Rethinking the universalism versus targeting debate," *Brookings,* May 31, 2017. brookings.edu/blog/future-development/2017/05/31/rethinking-the-universalism-versus-targeting-debate/; Quiñonez, *The Politics of Dental Care in Canada,* figures 2.18, 2.22.

108. Margaret Little, "A litmus test for democracy: The impact of Ontario welfare changes on single mothers," *Studies in Political Economy,* 66, 1 (2001): 9–36; "Is welfare a dirty word? Canadian public opinion on social assistance policies," *Policy Options,* September 1, 2008. policyoptions.irpp.org/fr/magazines/canadas-working-poor/is-welfare-a-dirty-word-

canadian-public-opinion-on-social-assistance-policies/;
Wendy Chan, "Canada: Punishing the undeserving poor," *Open Democracy*, August 1, 2011. opendemocracy.net/en/5050/canada-punishing-undeserving-poor/.

109. Ross Finnie, Ian Irvine and Roger Sceviour, *Social assistance use in Canada: National and provincial trends in incidence, entry and exit,* Statistics Canada: Analytical Studies Branch Research Paper Series, 11, 245 (May 2005) 5.

110. Quiñonez, "The political economy of dentistry," 163–164.

111. Quiñonez, "The political economy of dentistry," 163.

112. Quiñonez, "The political economy of dentistry," 113, 206.

113. Quiñonez, "The political economy of dentistry," 226.

114. Shaw, *An Environmental Scan.*

115. Quiñonez, "Canadian dentists' opinions on publicly financed."

116. Quiñonez, "Canadian dentists' opinions on publicly financed."

117. "Take a bite out of inequality: The case for universal dental care," *Spring Magazine*, July 29, 2020. springmag.ca/take-a-bite-out-of-inequality-the-case-for-universal-dental-care; Mosby, "Federal policies undermine Indigenous dental health."

118. Robert Devet, "Dental care for people on income assistance a bit of a horror story," *Nova Scotia Advocate*, May 7, 2019. nsadvocate.org/2019/05/07/dental-care-for-people-on-income-assistance-a-bit-of-a-horror-story/.

119. Devet, "Dental care for people on income assistance."

120. Quiñonez, "The political economy of dentistry," 164.

121. Quiñonez, "The political economy of dentistry," 164.

122. Canadian Dental Association, "Dentures." cda-adc.ca/en/oral_health/procedures/bridges_dentures/dentures.asp.

123. Lange, "Comprehensive dental care in Canada."

124. Mario Brondani, Bruce Wallace and Leeann R. Donnelly, "Dental insurance and treatment patterns at a not-for-profit community dental clinic," *Journal of the Canadian Dental Association,* 85, 10 (2019).

125. Atlas of Public Management, "Targeted vs. universal programs," December 12, 2018. atlas101.ca/pm/concepts/targeted-vs-universal-programs/; Brandon Doucet, "It is time to implement a universal dental plan," *Toronto Star,* January 7, 2019. thestar.com/

opinion/contributors/2019/01/07/it-is-time-to-implement-a-universal-dental-plan.html.

126. Quiñonez, "The politics of dental care," fig. 3.16; Danyaal Raza, "Canada has a health-care investment problem," *Policy Options*, October 21, 2021. policyoptions.irpp.org/magazines/october-2021/canada-has-a-health-care-investment-problem/.

127. Statistics Canada: Health Fact Sheets, "Primary health care providers, 2019," October 22, 2020. 150.statcan.gc.ca/n1/pub/82-625-x/2020001/article/00004-eng.htm.

128. Lange, "Comprehensive dental care in Canada," 1.

129. Mark Merryfield, "A survey of periodontal conditions in adolescents enrolled in the Saskatchewan Health Dental Plan," Saskatchewan Health Dental Plan, (1983).

130. Stephanie Rezansoff, "SHDP: An experiment in success that failed," *Saskatchewan Economics Journal* (1997): 1–9.

131. Rezansoff, "SHDP: An experiment."

132. CCPA, "Putting our money whereout mouth is," 9, 41.

133. Quiñonez, "The political economy of dentistry," 151; Gary Ewart, "The Saskatchewan Children's Dental Plan: Is it time for renewal?" (dissertation, University of Regina, 2010): 77; Saskatchewan New Democratic Party, Campaign Literature, "Allan Blakeney and the NDP: Tested and trusted" (1982).

134. Rezansoff, "SHDP: An experiment": table 2.

135. Rezansoff, "SHDP: An experiment": table 1.

136. Carlos Quiñonez, "Why was dental care excluded"; Hasan Sheikh and Brandon Doucet, "Honour Tommy Douglas and stand up for public denticare," *Policy Options* (2022); Brandon Doucet, "Whatever happened to dental therapy in Canada," *Canadian Dimension* (2020).

137. CCPA, "Putting our money where our mouth is"; Quiñonez, "Dentistry in Alberta"; Canadian Association of Public Health Dentistry, "Roadmap to universal dental care in Canada: Submission to the House of Commons Standing Committee on Health" (September 9, 2020). https://caphd.ca/wp-content/uploads/2022/06/HOC_Universalaccess_Sep9-2020_fin.pdf.

Chapter 5: Benefiting from the Status Quo

1.   "Corporate dentistry: An alternative to individually-owned practices," *Juriscorp Law*. juriscorplaw.ca/corporate-dentistry-alternative-individually-owned-practices/.

2.   Chris Hannay, "Inside the corporate dash to buy up dentists' offices, veterinary clinics and pharmacies," *Globe and Mail* (2022). theglobeandmail.com/business/article-private-equity-buy-out-pharmacy-dental-office-veterinary-clinic/.

3.   Group Dentistry Now, "Largest majority Canadian-owned network of dental practice poised for more national expansion," May 27, 2020. groupdentistrynow.com/dso-group-blog/largest-majority-canadian-owned-network-of-dental-practices-poised-for-more-national-expansion/.

4.   Nick Korhonen, "Practice models," Dental Career Options. https://dentalcareeroptions.ca/practice-models/.

5.   "123Dentist and Altima dental announce a strategic merger with support from Peloton Capital, KKR, and Heartland Dental," *Businesswire* (2022). businesswire.com/news/home/20220712005258/en/123Dentist-and-Altima-Dental-Announce-a-Strategic-Merger-with-Support-from-Peloton-Capital-KKR-and-Heartland-Dental.

6.   Oral Health Group, "Dentalcorp celebrates successful beginnings," July 5, 2017.

7.   "Dentalcorp reports strong second quarter 2021 results," *Newswire*, August 10, 2021. www.newswire.ca/news-releases/dentalcorp-reports-strong-second-quarter-2021-results-877936976.html.

8.   Hannay, "Inside the corporate dash"; "Dentalcorp and Loblaw Companies Ltd. bring digital dental health services to Canadians," *Newswire*, August 9, 2021. newswire.ca/news-releases/dentalcorp-and-loblaw-companies-ltd-bring-digital-dental-health-services-to-canadians-863334748.html; Bethany Lindsay, "Corporations swallow up BC dental practices," *Vancouver Sun*, April 26, 2016. vancouversun.com/news/local-news/corporations-swallow-up-b-c-dental-practices.

9.   Hannay, "Inside the corporate dash."

10. Group Dentistry Now, "Private equity reinforces its investment

with Canadian dental group," October 2, 2019. groupdentistrynow. com/dso-group-blog/private-equity-reinforces-its-investment-with-canadian-dental-group/.

11. CDA (Canadian Dental Association), "Economic realities of practice." Cda-adc.ca/en/services/internationallytrained/economic/.

12. Hannay, "Inside the corporate dash."

13. David Heath, Mark Greenblatt and Aysha Bagchi, "Dentists under pressure to drill 'healthy teeth' for profit, former insiders allege," *USA Today*, March 19, 2020. usatoday.com/in-depth/news/investigations/2020/03/19/dental-chain-private-equity-drills-healthy-teeth-profit/4536783002/.

14. Michael Carabash, "Rise of the DSOs (Dental Service Organizations) in Canada," *DMC Dentist Lawyers*, June 20, 2017. dentistlawyers.ca/rise-dsos-dental-service-organizations-canada/.

15. "Dentalcorp Completes US $908 Million Debt Financing," *Newswire*, June 7, 2018. newswire.ca/news-releases/dentalcorp-completes-us-908-million-debt-financing-684847061.html.

16. Group Dentistry Now, "Largest majority Canadian-owned."

17. David Heath, "Dental boards rarely punish dentists for unnecessary treatment," *USA Today News*, March 19, 2020. usatoday.com/in-depth/news/investigations/2020/03/19/dental-board-rarely-suspend-dentist-license-bad-dentistry/5014443002/.

18. Ake Blomqvist and Frances Woolley, *Filling the cavities. Improving the efficiency and equity of Canada's dental care system*, CD Howe Institute Commentary 510 (2018).

19. CDA "Economic realities of practice."

20. Group Dentistry Now, "Largest majority Canadian-owned."

21. David Burger, "Dental companies agree to $5.1 million settlement for alleged fraud," *ADA News*, November 13, 2018.

22. Ferris Jabr, Laura Marsh and Alex Pareene, "More reasons to hate the dentist," *New Republic*, July 21, 2021. newrepublic.com/article/163012/reasons-hate-dentist-malpractice.

23. Office of the Attorney General Press Release Archives, "A.G. Schneiderman announces settlement with Aspen Dental Management that bars company from making decisions about patient care in new york clinics," June 18, 2015. ag.ny.gov/

press-release/2015/ag-schneiderman-announces-settlement-aspen-dental-management-bars-company-making.

24.   David Heath and Jill Rosenbaum, "Patients, pressure and profits at Aspen Dental," PBS *Frontline*, June 26, 2012. pbs.org/wgbh/frontline/article/patients-pressure-and-profits-at-aspen-dental/; United States Attorney's Office Western District of Kentucky, "$5.1 million dollar settlement reached with Indiana dental firm to resolve false claims allegations," November 6, 2018. justice.gov/usao-wdky/pr/51-million-dollar-settlement-reached-indiana-dental-firm-resolve-false-claims.

25.   Heath, "Dental boards rarely punish."

26.   Jabr, "More reasons to hate the dentist."

27.   Cheryl Bell, "Newly named dentalcorp Simulation Lab: A training ground for oral health care professionals," *Dal News*, April 29, 2019. dal.ca/news/2019/04/29/newly-named-dentalcorp-simulation-lab--a-training-ground-for-ora.html; Dentalcorp, "$1-million gift from dentalcorp helps Western advance the future of dentistry," September 26, 2019. dentalcorp.ca/site/blog/2019/09/26/1-million-gift-helps-western-advance-the-future-of-dentistry; Dentalcorp, "Dentalcorp donates largest gift in USask College of Dentistry history," September 12, 2019. dentalcorp.ca/site/blog/2019/09/12/dentalcorp-donates-largest-gift-in-usask-college-of-dentistry-history.

28.   "Canada's universities and colleges are being taken over by big corporations and wealthy donors," *Press Progress*, January 31, 2019. pressprogress.ca/canadas-universities-and-colleges-are-being-taken-over-by-big-corporations-and-wealthy-donors/.

29.   Dentalcorp, "Dental Corporation Commits $250,000 to Paediatric Dentistry in Canada," September 15, 2014. globenewswire.com/news-release/2014/09/15/1431986/0/en/Dental-Corporation-Commits-250-000-to-Paediatric-Dentistry-in-Canada.html.

30.   University of New Brunswick, "Tax incentives." unb.ca/giving/impact/taxincentives.html.

31.   Tracey Adams, *A Dentist and a Gentleman: Gender and the Rise of Dentistry in Ontario* (Toronto: University of Toronto Press, 2000): 73.

32.   SmileDirectClub, "Here's how it works." smiledirectclub.ca/en-ca/how_it_works/.

33. Jenny Cowley, David Common and Jeannie Stiglic, "Hidden camera investigation finds misleading information, questionable treatment plans from SmileDirectClub," CBC *Marketplace*, March 28, 2020. cbc.ca/news/canada/hidden-camera-investigation-finds-misleading-information-questionable-treatment-plans-from-smiledirectclub-1.5511095.

34. Cowley, "Hidden camera investigation finds misleading information"; Saleh Daghreeer, "Invisalign vs. Braces cost in Canada," *City Orthodontics & Pediatric Dentistry*, October 4, 2021. cityorthopeds.com/2021/10/invisalign-vs-braces-cost-in-canada/.

35. Cowley, "Hidden camera investigation finds misleading information."

36. Nabeel Talic, "Adverse effects of orthodontic treatment: A clinical perspective," *Saudi Dental Journal*, 23, 2 (2011): 55–59.

37. Cowley, "Hidden camera investigation finds misleading information."

38. Caitlyn Gowrilukm, "Teeth-straightening company files 1st lawsuit in Canada against Manitoba dental group," CBC *News*, August 30, 2019.

39. "SmileDirectClub partners with leading dental insurer Green Shield Canada," *GlobalNewsWire*, January 27, 2021. globenewswire.com/news-release/2021/01/27/2165044/0/en/SmileDirectClub-Partners-With-Leading-Dental-Insurer-Green-Shield-Canada.html.

40. Michael Law, Jillian Kratzer and Irfan A. Dhalla, "The increasing inefficiency of private health insurance in Canada," *Canadian Medical Association Journal*, 186, 12 (2014): 470–E474.

41. Steffie Woolhandler, Terry Campbell and David U. Himmelstein, "Costs of health care administration in the United States and Canada," *New England Journal of Medicine*, 349, 8 (2003): 768–775.

42. Kip Sullivan, "How to think clearly about Medicare administrative costs: Data sources and measurement," *Journal of Health Politics, Policy and Law*, 38, 3 (2013): 479–504; Law, "The increasing inefficiency of private health insurance."

43. Law, "The increasing inefficiency of private health insurance," figure 1.

44. Law, "The increasing inefficiency of private health insurance," figure 3.

45. Abigail Abrams, "The U.S. spends $2,500 per person on health care administrative costs. Canada spends $550. Here's why," *Time*, January 6, 2020. time.com/5759972/health-care-administrative-costs/.

46. Meng Qingyue, Jia Liying and Yuan Beibei, *Cost-Sharing Mechanisms in Health Insurance Schemes: A Systematic Review*, Alliance for Health Policy and Systems Research, WHO (2011): 1–76. https://www.cchds.pku.edu.cn/docs/2018-06/20180605093159721013.

47. Oved Chown, Toby Heaps and Micheal Yow, "The high cost of low corporate taxes," *Toronto Star*, December 14, 2017. https://projects.thestar.com/canadas-corporations-pay-less-tax-than-you-think/.

48. Carlos Quiñonez, "The political economy of dentistry in Canada" (doctoral dissertation, University of Toronto, 2009): 16–17; Mark Stabile, "Private insurance subsidies and public health care markets: Evidence from Canada," *Canadian Journal of Economics*, 34, 4 (2001): 921–942.

49. Stabile, "Private insurance subsidies"; Yves Giroux, "Cost estimate of a federal dental care program for uninsured Canadians," Office of the Parliamentary Budget Officer (2020): 8.

50. Quiñonez, "The political economy of dentistry," 16–17.

51. Osler, "New Canada Revenue Agency Position on Barbados Exempt Insurance Companies," November 12, 2010.

52. Sharon Batt, "The big money club: Revealing the players and their campaign to stop Pharmacare," Canadian Federation of Nurses Unions (2019).

53. Catharine Tunney, "Liberals agree to launch dental care program in exchange for NDP support," *CBC News* (2022). cbc.ca/news/politics/trudeu-jagmeet-singh-deal-government-1.6393021.

54. "Promises, promises," *Globe and Mail* (2004). theglobeandmail.com/news/national/promises-promises/article18265640/; Steve Morgan, "Universal public drug coverage would save Canada billions," University of British Columbia. spph.ubc.ca/universal-public-drug-coverage-would-save-canada-billions/

55. Batt, "The big money club," 10.

56. Batt, "The big money club," 10.

57. Batt, "The big money club," 18.

58.   Batt, "The big money club," 20.

59.   Mariana Mazzucato, "State of innovation: Busting the private-sector myth," *New Scientist*, August 21, 2013. newscientist.com/article/mg21929310-200-state-of-innovation-busting-the-private-sector-myth/; Theodore Eickhoff, "Penicillin: An accidental discovery changed the course of medicine," *Healio: Endocrinology*, August 10, 2008. healio.com/news/endocrinology/20120325/penicillin-an-accidental-discovery-changed-the-course-of-medicine; Ken Mactaggart, "It's penicillin," *Macleans*, December 1, 1943. archive.macleans.ca/article/1943/12/1/its-penicillin.

60.   Eickhoff, "Penicillin: An accidental discovery."

61.   John Nathan, Lynda Asadourian and Mark Erlich, "A brief history of local anesthesia," *International Journal of Head and Neck Surgery*, 7, 1 (Winter 2016): 29–32.

62.   Tae-Il Kim, "A tribute to Dr. Per-Ingvar Brånemark," *Journal of Periodontal Implant Science*, 44: 6 (2014) 265; Himed, "Titanium, rabbits, and tiny microscopes: Dr. Brånemark's unlikely discovery of the modern dental implant" (2021). himed.com/blog/origin-of-osseointegration-titanium-dental-implant.

63.   Congressional Budget Office, "Research and development in the pharmaceutical industry," April 2021. cbo.gov/publication/57126.

64.   Mazzucato, "State of innovation."

Chapter 6: The Future of Dental Care in Canada

1.   "Know the drill: What Canadians need to know about dental tourism," CTV *News*, February 19, 2018. bc.ctvnews.ca/know-the-drill-what-canadians-need-to-know-about-dental-tourism-1.3810334.

2.   Daniela Neumann and Carlos Quiñonez, "A comparative analysis of oral health care systems in the United States, United Kingdom, France, Canada, and Brazil," NCOHR *Working Paper Series* 1 (2014): 1–18.

3.   Seán Boyle, "United Kingdom (England): Health system review," *World Health Organization* (2011); J. Winkelmann, C. Henschke, S. Scarpetti and D. Panteli, "Dental care in Europe: Financing, coverage and provision," *European Journal of Public Health*, 30, 5

(2020): 165–985.

4.	I am Expat, "Dental care in Germany." iamexpat.de/expat-info/german-healthcare-system/dental-care-germany; Sara Allin, Julie Farmer, Carlos Quiñonez, Allie Peckham, Gregory Marchildon, Dimitra Panteli and Cornelia Henschke, "Do health systems cover the mouth? Comparing dental care coverage for older adults in eight jurisdictions," *Health Policy,* 124, 9 (2020): 998–1007.

5.	Anna Sagan and Sarah Thomson, "Voluntary health insurance in Europe: Role and regulation," European Observatory on Heath Systems and Policies (2016). https://www.euro.who.int/__data/assets/pdf_file/0005/310838/Voluntary-health-insurance-Europe-role-regulation.pdf.

6.	Henri Lewalle, "A look at private health care insurance in the European Union," *Revue Française des affaires sociales* (2006): 133–157.

7.	Neumann, "A comparative analysis of oral health care systems," table 3.

8.	Claire Wilde, "NHS dentistry 'hanging by a thread' after nearly 1,000 dentists quit service," *National World,* January 21, 2022. nationalworld.com/news/uk/nhs-dentistry-hanging-by-a-thread-after-nearly-1000-dentists-quit-service-3536350; Neumann, "A comparative analysis of oral health care systems," table 4.

9.	Amanda Biggs, "Dental reform: An overview of universal dental schemes," Department of Parliamentary Services: Australian Government (2012): 5.

10.	Susan Moffat, Lyndie Page and Murray Thomson, "New Zealand's school dental service over the decades: Its response to social, political, and economic influences, and the effect on oral health inequalities," *Frontiers in Public Health,* 5 (2017): 177.

11.	Tai-Yin Wu, Azeem Majeed and Ken N. Kuo, "An overview of the healthcare system in Taiwan," *London Journal of Primary Care* 3, 2 (2010): 115–119; Takashi Zaitsu, Tomoya Saito and Yoko Kawaguchi, "The oral healthcare system in Japan," *Healthcare MDPI,* 6, 3 (July 2018): 79.

12.	United Nations Development Group, "Theory of change: UNDAF Companion Guidance" (2017). https://unsdg.un.org/resources/theory-change-undaf-companion-guidance.

13. Anjum Sultana and Jacquie Maund, "Needed: A Tommy Douglas for dental care," Alliance for Healthier Communities, May 14, 2015. allianceon.org/news/Needed-Tommy-Douglas-Dental-Care.

14. "Ontario NDP dental plan to cost $1.2 billion," *City News*, March 19, 2018. toronto.citynews.ca/2018/03/19/ontario-ndp-dental-plan/; Kristin Rushowy, "Andrea Horwath says NDP would provide dental care plan for low- and middle-income Ontarians," *Toronto Star* (2022). thestar.com/politics/provincial/2022/05/05/ndp-leader-andrea-horwath-promising-dental-care-plan-that-works-with-federal-one-if-elected.html.

15. Jeff Semple, "Canadians support publicly funded dental care for those without insurance, Ipsos poll finds," *Global News*, May 14, 2019. globalnews.ca/news/5273773/canadians-support-publicly-funded-dental-care-for-those-without-insurance-poll-finds/.

16. Alex Marland, "Why minority governments have been good — and sometimes bad — for Canada," The Conversation, September 23, 2021. theconversation.com/why-minority-governments-have-been-good-and-sometimes-bad-for-canada-168018.

17. Tom Kent, "When minority government worked: The Pearson legacy," *Policy Options*, October 1, 2009. policyoptions.irpp.org/magazines/minority-government/when-minority-government-worked-the-pearson-legacy/.

18. Geoff Norquay, "Minority governments considered: Are they the new normal?" *Policy Options*, October 1, 2009. policyoptions.irpp.org/fr/magazines/minority-government/minority-governments-considered-are-they-the-new-normal/.

19. Rachel Aiello, "Liberals, NDP have tentative deal that would keep Trudeau government in power until 2025," *CTV News*, March 21, 2022. https://www.ctvnews.ca/politics/liberals-ndp-have-tentative-deal-that-would-keep-trudeau-government-in-power-until-2025-1.5828863.

20. Catharine Tunney, "Liberals agree to launch dental care program in exchange for NDP support," *CBC News*, March 22, 2022. https://www.cbc.ca/news/politics/trudeu-jagmeet-singh-deal-government-1.6393021.

21. Nick Boisvert, "Everything we know about the Liberal–NDP dental care proposal," *CBC News*, March 23, 2022. https://www.cbc.ca/

news/politics/liberal-ndp-dental-plan-1.6393981.

22. Diarra Sourang and Aidan Worswick, "Cost estimate of a federal dental care program for uninsured Canadians," Office of the Parliamentary Budget Officer, October 7, 2020; Government of Canada, "Chapter 6: Strong Public Health Care," April 7, 2022. budget.gc.ca/2022/report-rapport/chap6-en.html; Government of Canada, "Message from the Minister of Health regarding request for information from industry on proposed national dental care program" (2022). canada.ca/en/health-canada/news/2022/07/message-from-the-minister-of-health-regarding-request-for-information-from-industry-on-proposed-national-dental-care-program.html.

23. Ed Broadbent and Libby Davies, "How the NDP can effect change in a minority government," CBC Radio, October 25, 2019. cbc.ca/radio/sunday/the-sunday-edition-for-october-27-2019-1.5335017/how-the-ndp-can-effect-change-in-a-minority-government-1.5335027.

24. Rebecca Gao, "What a 'Vote of no confidence' means in Canadian politics," Readers Digest, February 22, 2022. readersdigest.ca/culture/vote-of-no-confidence/.

25. Chelsea Nash, "Broadbent says NDP 'should be worried' Liberals won't live up to commitments in upcoming budget, must keep pressure on," Hill Times, April 3, 2022. hilltimes.com/2022/04/03/broadbent-says-ndp-should-be-worried-liberals-wont-live-up-to-commitments-in-upcoming-budget-must-keep-pressure-on/353519.

26. Anja Karadeglija, "Battle over a national dental care plan looming with provinces," National Post, April 20, 2022. nationalpost.com/news/politics/battle-over-a-national-dental-care-plan-looming-with-provinces.

27. Walter Korpi and Joakim Palme, "The paradox of redistribution and strategies of equality: welfare state institutions, inequality and poverty in the western countries," American Sociological Review, 63, 5 (1998): 22.

28. Garry Ewart, "The Saskatchewan Children's Dental Plan: Is it time for renewal?" (dissertation, University of Regina, 2010).

29. Andrea Hill, "Relaunch of a dental therapy program in Sask. would

address needs of First Nations," *Saskatoon StarPheonix*, March 29, 2021. thestarphoenix.com/news/local-news/relaunch-of-a-dental-therapy-program-in-sask-would-address-needs-of-first-nations; "USask collaboration establishes first dental therapy degree program in Canada," *University of Saskatchewan* (2022). news.usask.ca/articles/colleges/2022/usask-collaboration-establishes-first-dental-therapy-degree-program-in-canada.php.

30. Canadian Dental Hygienists Association, "CDHA position statement: Filling the gap in oral health care" (July 2017): 2.

31. International Dentists Canada. "10 frequently asked questions by internationally trained dentists who wants to practice dentistry in Canada." internationaldentistscanada.com/10-frequently-asked-questions-by-internationally-trained-dentists-who-wants-to-practice-dentistry-in-canada/.

32. University of Toronto Faculty of Dentistry, "The international dentist advanced placement program (IDAPP)." dentistry.utoronto.ca/prospective-students/international-dentists/join-DDS-IDAPP.

33. DAT Crusher, "Dental schools costs in Canada." datcrusher.ca/classroom/admission-guide/dental-school-costs-in-canada/.

34. Government of Canada, "Dental Officer." forces.ca/en/career/dental officer/.

35. Christine Saulnier, "Many dangers of public-private partnerships (P3s) in Newfoundland and Labrador," Canadian Centre for Policy Alternatives (2020).

36. Chris Hannay, "Inside the corporate dash to buy up dentists' offices, veterinary clinics and pharmacies." *Globe and Mail* (2022). https://www.theglobeandmail.com/business/article-private-equity-buy-out-pharmacy-dental-office-veterinary-clinic/.

37. Stan Rands, *Privilege and Policy: A History of Community Clinics in Saskatchewan, Revised Edition* (Edmonton: Canadian Plains Research Centre Press, 2012): 89.

38. Rands, *Privilege and Policy*, 89.

39. Rands, *Privilege and Policy*, 79–89.

40. Carlos Quiñonez, Rafael Figueiredo and David Locker, "Canadian dentists' opinions on publicly financed dental care," *Journal of Public Health Dentistry*, 69, 2 (2009): table 5; Semple, "Canadians support publicly funded dental care."

41. Jamie Moeller and Carlos Quiñonez, "The association between income inequality ad oral health in Canada: A cross-sectional study," *International Journal of Health Services*, October 2016; "The high cost of food on First Nations reserves," *TVO Current Affairs*, January 19, 2017. tvo.org/article/the-high-cost-of-food-on-first-nations-reserves; Leyland Cecco, "Dozens of Canada's First Nations lack clean drinking water: 'Unacceptable in a country so rich," *Guardian*, April 30, 2021. theguardian.com/world/2021/apr/30/canada-first-nations-justin-trudeau-drinking-water; Peter Zimonjic, "Health care system was designed to subject Indigenous people to systemic racism: Hajdu," *CBC News*, October 15, 2020. cbc.ca/news/politics/health-indigenous-racism-miller-1.5764659; Anne Kingston, "How bad teeth are at the root of income inequality in Canada," *Maclean's*, November 6, 2017. macleans.ca/society/how-bad-teeth-are-at-the-root-of-income-inequality-in-canada/.

42. Oxfam Canada, "10 richest men double their fortunes in pandemic while incomes of 99 per cent of humanity fall," January 16, 2022. oxfam.ca/news/10-richest-men-double-their-fortunes-in-pandemic-while-incomes-of-99-per-cent-of-humanity-fall/.

43. Alex Hemingway, "Robust wealth tax could raise $363B over 10 years," *Policy Note*, September 14, 2021. policynote.ca/federal-wealth-tax/. Canadian Union of Public Employees, "New report shows Canadian companies are keeping $381 billion in offshore tax havens," July 22, 2020. cupe.ca/new-report-shows-canadian-companies-are-keeping-381-billion-offshore-tax-havens.

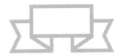

INDEX